Handbook of Hip Fracture Surgery

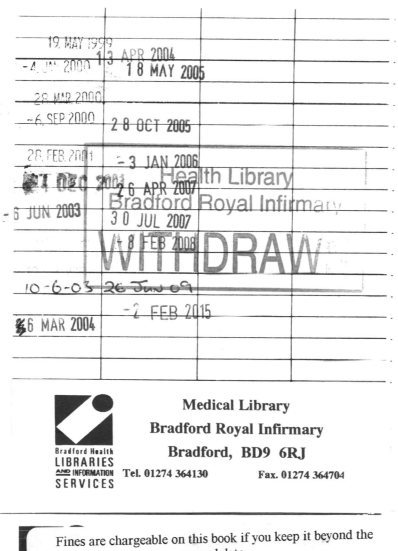

Handbook of Hip Fracture Surgery

Martyn J Parker MD, FRCS (Edin)
Orthopaedic Research Fellow
Peterborough District Hospital
Peterborough, UK

Glyn A Pryor MS, FRCS
Consultant Orthopaedic Surgeon
Peterborough District Hospital
Peterborough, UK

Karl-Göran Thorngren MD
Professor of Orthopaedic Surgery
Lund University Hospital
Lund
Sweden

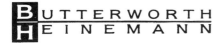

Butterworth-Heinemann
Linacre House, Jordan Hill, Oxford OX2 8DP
A division of Reed Educational and Professional Publishing Ltd

Ɫ A member of the Reed Elsevier plc group

OXFORD   BOSTON   JOHANNESBURG
MELBOURNE   NEW DELHI   SINGAPORE

First published 1997

British Library Cataloguing in Publication Data
A catalogue record for this book is available from the British Library

Library of Congress Cataloging in Publication Data
A catalogue record for this book is available from the Library of Congress

ISBN 0 7506 2179 6

Set by Interactive Sciences Ltd, Gloucester
Printed and bound in Great Britain by The Bath Press

Contents

Preface   vii

1   Epidemiology of proximal femoral fracture   1

2   Diagnosis, fracture classification and treatment options   7

3   Patient assessment and initial management   29

4   Use of the fracture table and image intensifier   39

5   Internal fixation of intracapsular fractures   45

6   Extramedullary fixation of extracapsular fractures   63

7   Intramedullary fixation of extracapsular fractures   91

8   Arthroplasty   111

9   Postoperative care   133

Index   141

Preface

This book aims to give practical instruction for the trainee orthopaedic surgeon in what is probably the commonest fracture he or she will encounter. The operative treatment of proximal femoral fractures is often left to the orthopaedic trainee, even though fixation of comminuted fractures in osteoporotic bone can present a formidable challenge to even the most experienced surgeon.

The emphasis is on the practical details of surgery and general management. This is not intended as a comprehensive reference book, and suggested reading gives information on more detailed texts.

1

Epidemiology of proximal femoral fracture

An increasingly aged population presents two challenges to orthopaedic and trauma services – osteoarthritic joints and osteoporotic fractures. Replacement arthroplasty for arthritic joints has been the great success story in orthopaedics over the past 30 years. However, in parallel with the rising demand for elective arthroplasty, increasing numbers of elderly trauma patients have been presenting with an osteoporotic fracture. The hip, vertebrae and distal radius are the commonest sites of osteoporotic fractures; of these, it is the hip which is associated with the greatest mortality and morbidity.

The incidence of proximal femoral fracture

The rising number of proximal femoral fractures is well-documented worldwide. Probably about half of all such fractures occur in Europe and North America (Table 1.1).

The incidence of proximal femoral fracture rises exponentially with age (Fig. 1.1). This increase becomes significant from the age of 60 years in women and later in men. By the age of 90 years a woman has a 1 in 20 chance of suffering a hip fracture each year. The lifetime risk for a woman is 15%, compared to 5% for a man.

Table 1.1 Reported annual incidence of hip fractures from different countries per 100 000 of population (Parker and Pryor, 1993)

Country	Number
Sweden	165
Canada	103
Finland	91
UK	86
USA	80
Malaysia	70
Israel	59
Korea	34

The rising number of fractures is not only due to the increasing longevity of the population. More alarmingly, there appears to be a rise in the age-specific incidence, particularly in those over 80 years of age. However, there is some uncertainty as to whether this rising incidence, which was apparent up to the 1980s, is still occurring (Fig. 1.2).

Regardless of a rise in the true incidence, the demographic changes occurring in all populations throughout the world will lead to a dramatic increase in hip fractures over the next 30 years.

The most important factors influencing the incidence are age and sex. There is also considerable racial variation, with Caucasian

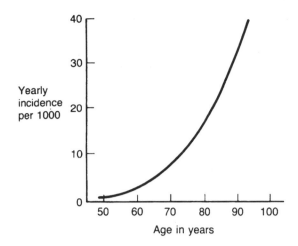

Fig. 1.1   Incidence of hip fracture related to age. From Cummings SR, Nevitt MC. A hypothesis: the causes of hip fracture. *J Gerontol* 1989; **44**:107–111, with permission.

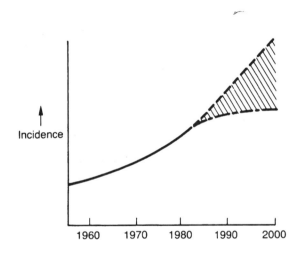

Fig. 1.2   Previous and predicted increase (shaded area) in the incidence of hip fractures.

populations having the highest rate and Negroes of South Africa the lowest reported incidence. Genetic factors are likely to be the reason for these differences. Higher bone mass is probably the main reason for the lower rate amongst Negroes. Incidence rates vary within countries, with rural populations having lower age-specific rates than urban ones.

There are geographic variations in fracture incidence, with a rising risk further from the Equator. This has been suggested to be due to the influence of sunlight on vitamin D synthesis. Seasonal variation and nutritional factors have been reported by some authors, but this is not a universal finding. Smoking, alcohol, a variety of drugs, particularly corticosteroids, and a number of medical conditions have also been found to be associated with increased risk of hip fracture.

The causes of hip fracture

Alffram in the early 1960s first elucidated the cause of these fractures as an interplay of three factors – age, disease and trauma. The majority are due to a combination of age-related factors, principally age-related bone loss, and trauma, which is generally a minor fall.

More recently, other authors have expanded on the precise mechanism by which these fractures occur. The clearest explanation is given by Cummings and Nevitt (1989), who proposed the following hypothesis to explain how a hip fracture is caused. Most hip fractures are caused by a fall from standing height; however, to cause a fracture, the following conditions must be satisfied. The person falling must land on or near the hip; protective responses must be inadequate to reduce the energy of the fall; local shock absorbers must be inadequate to absorb the energy; and bone strength must be insufficient to resist the residual energy of the fall (Fig. 1.3).

This excellent hypothesis explains very well the increasing incidence of hip fracture with age. The steps act in a cascade fashion, with each factor following on from the next to multiply the chances of the fracture occurring. Table 1.2 lists some of the factors associated with an increased risk of sustaining a hip fracture.

Elderly people have a slower walking speed. The normal 60-year-old person who trips and cannot avoid falling will have sufficient impulsion to fall forward on to his or her hands. If a fracture occurs it is more likely to be of the distal radius. An 80 year old, in contrast, moving slowly, will tend to collapse down, landing to one side or the other, close to the hip (Fig. 1.4). The speed of protective

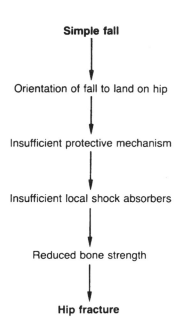

Simple fall

↓

Orientation of fall to land on hip

↓

Insufficient protective mechanism

↓

Insufficient local shock absorbers

↓

Reduced bone strength

↓

Hip fracture

Fig. 1.3 Factors implicated in the aetiology of a hip fracture. From Cummings SR, Nevitt MC. A hypothesis: the causes of hip fracture. *J Gerontol* 1989; **44**:107–111.

responses will decrease with age, as does the muscle mass around the hip. Bone mineral content, and hence its strength, diminishes with age and hence the residual fall energy is more likely to exceed the fracture threshold.

The fracture threshold is an abstract term referring to the strength of osteoporotic bone and the level below which fractures will occur with little or no trauma. As bone mass measurement techniques – essentially densiometry – have become more widespread, objective measurements of bone mineral density should be used to describe bone strength. However, it must be emphasized that the strength of bone depends on its structure as well as its mass or density.

Vertebral bodies are largely composed of cancellous bone. Age-related bone loss leads to a progressive reduction in trabeculae, especially the horizontal ones bracing the cube-like vertebral structure. Eventually the vertebra fails under compressive loading and collapses – a vertebral compression fracture.

The situation in the proximal femur is more complex. The femoral neck is largely cortical bone, while the trochanteric region contains

Table 1.2 Factors that have been implicated in the aetiology of hip fractures

Factors related to an increased risk of falls
Increased age

Concurrent medical illness

Drugs – tranquillizers, alcohol, antihypertensives

Senile dementia or confusional states

Physical disabilities or walking difficulties

Lack of regular exercise

Visual impairment

Cardiac arrhythmias and cardiac disease

Parkinson's disease and other neuromuscular diseases

Electrolyte imbalance

Hypothermia

Factors related to reduction in protective responses
Progressive decline with age

Senile dementia or confusional states

Muscle weakness or neuromuscular disorder

Factors related to loss of local shock absorbers
Loss of fat and muscle from around the hip

Factors related to a reduction in bone strength
Drugs – corticosteroids, anticonvulsants, thyroxine, alcohol

Cigarette smoking

Lack of minerals (calcium, magnesium, fluoride)

Vitamin D deficiency

Physical inactivity – both in early life and later years

Immobility, e.g. following a stroke

Low body weight

Malnutrition and low calcium intake, e.g. after gastrectomy or small-bowel disease

White or Asian racial origin

Nulliparity

Late menarche

Early menopause

Oophorectomy

Parathyroid disease

Hyperthyroidism

Hypercortisolism

Hypogonadism

Chronic renal failure

Chronic liver disease

Malignant disease of bone

Paget's disease

Radiotherapy to the hip area

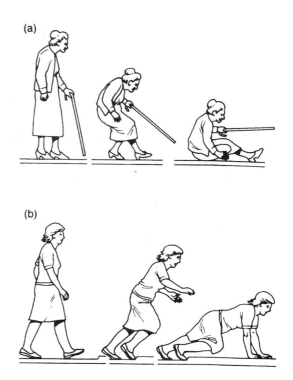

Fig. 1.4   Difference between a simple fall in (a) an elderly and (b) a younger person. From Cummings SR, Nevitt MC. A hypothesis: the causes of hip fracture. *J Gerontol* 1989; **44**:107–111, with permission.

roughly equal amounts of cancellous and cortical bone. Epidemiologically the proximal femoral fracture population may well contain different subgroups. Patients sustaining intracapsular fractures have in some studies been reported to have differing characteristics from those who suffer extracapsular fractures. Moreover, when a patient suffers a second fracture of the other hip, this is nearly always of the same type – intracapsular or extracapsular – as the first side.

Trabecular bone, of more relevance in trochanteric fractures, is more responsive to metabolic influences. This may be why certain individuals will be at greater risk of extracapsular fractures. Although bone loss can occur at any time during life, related to lifestyle, illness or drugs, the most important factor is the postmenopausal bone loss, related to lack of oestrogen. Hormone replacement therapy has been shown to exert a protective effect on bone, particularly preventing the loss that occurs following the menopause.

Hormone replacement therapy reduces fracture risk, especially vertebral compression fractures, in 50–65-year-old women. Its value in the older woman, who has already lost substantial bone, is less clear. Moreover, as the average age for a hip fracture is 80 years, it is uncertain whether the protective effect of hormone replacement therapy will persist until the period of maximum risk. Most women take hormone replacement therapy for only a short time; at least 5–10 years of treatment is required to achieve significant beneficial effects on the skeleton.

Other measures may be more important than hormone replacement therapy in the older woman. Drugs such as the bisphosphonates have been shown to reduce vertebral fracture rates and may be valuable in the older population who are at greatest risk of hip fracture. Other drugs, such as calcitonin and tamoxifen, may also have a protective effect, although they are still being investigated.

A French study of elderly nursing-home residents (Chapuy et al., 1994) found that vitamin D supplements reduced hip fracture rates. However, there has been considerable variation in the reported incidence of osteomalacia in hip fracture and other elderly populations. Certainly vitamin D and calcium supplements may well be of value in the institutionalized elderly.

The most important protective measures are lifestyle changes, diet and exercise, which have important influences throughout life. In the very old, exercise may maintain muscle mass and coordination. This can protect against the tendency to fall and thus reduce the fracture risk. In the discussion on drugs to prevent hip fractures it is important not to lose sight of other measures that are of fundamental value, especially in the very elderly who have already irretrievably lost most of their bone mass.

As well as the microstructure, the overall shape of the proximal femur may influence the strength and hence the fracture risk. A recent study from Reid et al. (1994) has reported that the length of the femoral neck in elderly women has increased over the past 40 years. This increase has been suggested to be the reason for the age-specific rise in hip fracture rate over this period. A torsional strain on a loaded femur will cause it to break at its weakest point, that is, the femoral neck, which is more horizontal. This is not a new observation and was recognized in case histories by Sir Astley Cooper over 150 years ago.

In summary, hip fractures are a major public health issue, especially in Northern European countries. The aetiology involves an interplay of age-related factors, osteoporosis and increased tendency to fall. The impact of these fractures will undoubtedly increase over the next decades, as the number of elderly in the population increases.

Key references and further reading

Alffram PA. An epidemiological study of cervical and trochanteric fractures of the femur in an urban population. *Acta Orthop Scand* 1964; Suppl 65.

Chapuy MC, Arlot ME, Delmas PD, Meunier PJ. Effect of calcium and cholecalciferol treatment for three years on hip fractures in elderly women. *Br Med J* 1994; **308**:1081–1082.

Cooper A. A treatise of dislocation and on fractures of the joints. Longman, Rees, London, 1822.

Cummings SR, Nevitt MC. A hypothesis: the causes of hip fracture. *J Gerontol* 1989; **44**:107–111.

Hollingworth W, Todd CJ, Parker MJ. The cost of treating hip fractures in the twenty-first century. *J Public Health* 1995; **17**:269–276.

Jarnlo G-B, Ceder L, Thorngren K-G. Early rehabilitation at home of elderly patients with hip fractures and consumption of resources in primary care. *Scand J Primary Health Care* 1984; **2**:105–112.

Jarnlo G-B, Thorngren K-G. Background factors to hip fractures. *Clin Orthop* 1993; **287**:41–49.

Law MR, Wald NJ, Meade TW. Strategies for prevention of osteoporosis and hip fracture. *Br Med J* 1991; **303**:453–459.

Newman RJ. *Orthogeriatrics: Comprehensive Care of the Elderly Patient*. Butterworth Heinemann, London, 1992.

NHS Centre for Reviews and Dissemination. University of York. Effective health care; Preventing falls and subsequent injury in older people. 1996; Vol 2:No 4.

Parker MJ, Pryor GA. *Hip Fracture Management*. Blackwell Scientific Publications, Oxford, 1993.

Practical aspects of the management of osteoporosis. *Int Med* 1986; suppl 12.

Reid IR, Chin K, Evans MC, Jones JG. Relation between increase in length of hip axis in older women between 1950s and 1990s and increase in age specific rates of hip fracture. *Br Med J* 1994; **309**:508–509.

Riggs BL, Melton LJ (eds). *Osteoporosis: Etiology, Diagnosis and Management*. Raven Press, New York, 1988.

Royal College of Physicians of London. *Fractured Neck of Femur: Prevention and Management*. Associated Book Publishers, London, 1989.

Thorngren K-G. Fractures in older persons. *Disability Rehabilitation* 1994; **16**:119–126.

Tinetti ME, Speechley M, Ginter SF. Risk factors for falls among elderly persons living in the community. *N Engl J Med* 1988; **319**:1701–1707.

Zetterberg C, Andersson GBJ. Fractures of the proximal end of the femur in Göteborg, Sweden, 1940–1979. *Acta Orthop Scand* 1982; **53**:419–426.

2

Diagnosis, fracture classification and treatment options

Diagnosis

Generally the diagnosis of a hip fracture is made without difficulty. The typical picture is that of an elderly female, who complains of a painful groin or thigh and being unable to rise or walk following a fall. Clinical signs are a shortened externally rotated limb with painful hip movements. In this situation X-ray of the hip will invariably confirm the diagnosis.

In up to 10% of cases the diagnosis may be delayed. This may be due to patient factors, such as mental impairment or previous poor mobility. There may occasionally be no history of a fall, with the fracture occurring spontaneously. In addition, if the fracture is undisplaced the clinical signs may be ambiguous. The patient will complain of mild to moderate pain and may be able to walk, albeit with difficulty. There will be no deformity of the limb and full passive movements of the hip may be possible. For the majority of these cases radiological signs are still apparent. A hip fracture with a completely normal radiograph is possible but very uncommon. If there is any doubt on reviewing the X-rays, the following features should be checked:

1 The anteroposterior (AP) view of the pelvis should be taken with both legs in 10° of internal rotation to enable comparison between each side.

2 A lateral view of the hip must always be obtained. Exposure of the film may need to be adjusted to obtain a clear view of the bone in the femoral neck.

3 In doubtful cases an additional AP view with the X-ray beam centred on the hip in question may be helpful. The exposure is adjusted to allow adequate detail to be shown in the femoral neck. In some situations this may require a different exposure to obtain clarity of detail within the trochanteric region.

4 AP and lateral views should be studied to determine if there is any break in continuity of the cortical margins, any change in the cortical bone appearance or distortion of the normal trabecular angle of 160° (Fig. 2.1).

Errors in diagnosis may occur with inadequate X-rays. Figure 2.2 illustrates an impacted intracapsular fracture with the leg in external rotation. The greater trochanter lies behind the femoral neck and obscures the fracture. Internally rotating the leg corrects this and the fracture becomes visible. Often a patient presenting with a hip fracture will have the affected leg in external rotation and the radiographer is often reluctant to rotate the limb internally through fear of causing pain.

The commonest type of fracture to be missed is the impacted intracapsular fracture

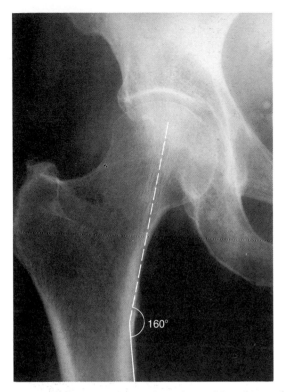

Fig. 2.1 The trabecular angle is formed by the angle between the trabeculae of the femoral head and shaft of the femur. It is normally 160° and can be measured on the normal hip to compare with that of the fractured side.

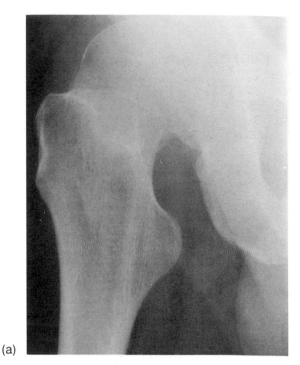

(a)

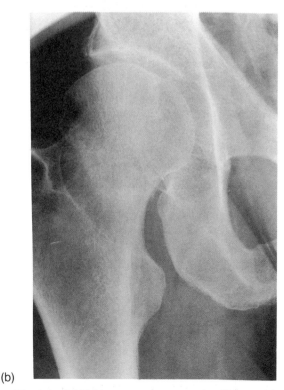

(b)

(Fig. 2.3). A crack fracture in the trochanteric region may also be overlooked (Fig. 2.4).

For the patient who complains of acute pain in the hip and in whom good-quality X-rays are normal, a number of options are available:

1 Allow the patient to mobilize as able. If a hip fracture is present the patient will complain of persistent pain and repeat X-rays will eventually confirm the fracture. There is however a risk that if a hip fracture is present, displacement will occur.

2 Keep the patient on bed rest for a period of 7–10 days and then repeat the hip X-rays or arrange X-ray tomography. If a fracture is present radiological signs should be present by this stage. This

Fig. 2.2 (a) Taking an anteroposterior X-ray with the hip in external rotation will obscure detail within the femoral neck. (b) Internally rotating the limb to 10° reveals an impacted intracapsular fracture.

(a)

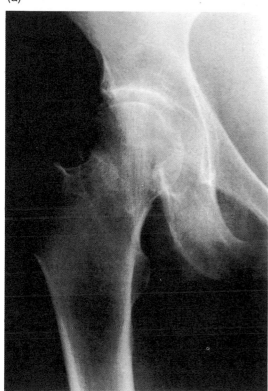

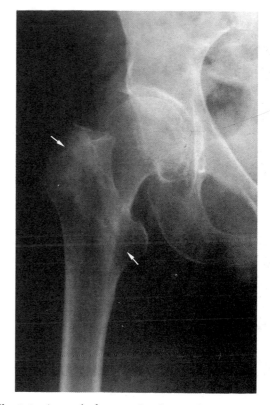

Fig. 2.4 A crack fracture in the trochanteric region (arrowed). The fracture may be missed if the X-ray exposure is not optimum.

(b)

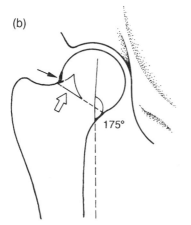

Fig. 2.3 (a) An impacted intracapsular fracture. The fracture can easily be missed. (b) Note the break in continuity of the lateral cortex at the neck (arrow) and an area of increased bone density at the site of impaction (open arrow). Lateral impaction results in an increase in the trabecular angle to 175°. Compare this with Figure 2.1, where the femoral neck is normal.

approach has now generally been super-seded by one of the investigations listed below.

3 Isotope bone scan will generally detect an occult fracture (Fig. 2.5). Difficulty in interpreting results may occur in the presence of arthritis of the hip or other inflammatory processes. Differentiating between an isolated fracture of the greater trochanter and a trochanteric fracture may also be difficult. The risk of a false-negative result may be reduced by either not performing the scan until a few days after injury, or by taking a delayed or 'pooled' scan image.

4 High-definition computed tomographic (CT) scanning of the hip may identify a fracture or the presence of haematoma with the hip joint. Experience of using CT scanning for the diagnosis of hip fractures is however limited.

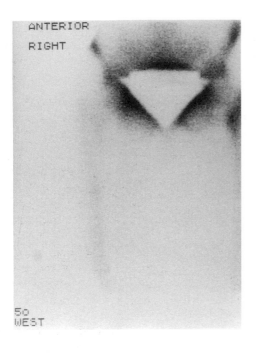

Fig. 2.5   Isotope bone scan demonstrating a trochanteric hip fracture.

5 A magnetic resonance imaging (MRI) scan will invariably demonstrate the fracture line. MRI appears to be more accurate than isotope bone scanning whilst being less invasive.

Classification of proximal femoral fractures

Fractures of the hip are classified based on the radiological appearance of the fracture. Incorrect interpretation of preoperative X-rays can have disastrous consequences necessitating repeat surgery, as illustrated in Figure 2.6.

Primary classification

The first and most important distinction is between intracapsular and extracapsular fractures. Intracapsular fractures are those which occur proximal to the attachment of the hip joint capsule. Extracapsular fractures occur in the region between the attachment of the

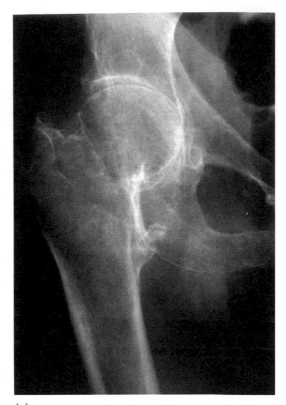

(a)

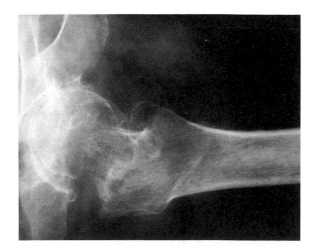

(b)

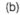

Fig. 2.6(a–c)   A trochanteric hip fracture. The X-rays were misinterpreted as an intracapsular fracture and the fracture treated with three parallel cancellous screws. Fixation failure was inevitable.

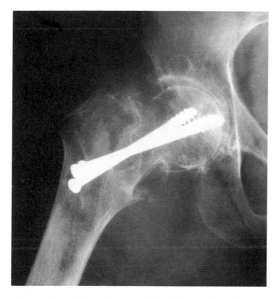

(c)

capsule and a line 5 cm distal to the lesser trochanter (Fig. 2.7).

Even this basic classification may lead to difficulties in interpretation. Basal fractures (Fig. 2.8) have a fracture line running along the line of the anterior attachment of the capsule. These fractures have previously been classified as both intracapsular and extra-capsular fractures. Their treatment and prognosis are more akin to an extracapsular fracture and it is best to consider these fractures as extracapsular.

Classification of intracapsular fractures

The terms subcapital and cervical are alternative names for this type of fracture. Strictly speaking, the term subcapital relates to intracapsular fractures running close to the articular surface. Cervical or transcervical fractures are those traversing the femoral neck. In clinical practice the distinction between these two fracture levels is ambiguous and of little clinical value. The terms cervical and subcapital have therefore become synonymous with the more precise term of intracapsular fracture.

The most important factor in the classification of intracapsular fractures is the prediction of healing complications, non-union and avascular necrosis. This should then serve to aid decision-making on whether internal fixation or primary arthroplasty is appropriate. Unfortunately, no such system exists and in practice many other factors will determine successful fracture healing.

Recommended classification

The simplest method of subdividing intracapsular fractures is the simple division into undisplaced and displaced fractures. For undisplaced intracapsular fractures expect an incidence of healing complications of 5–15% whilst for a displaced fracture the incidence is 15–35%.

The term undisplaced intracapsular fracture is used broadly to include impacted and minimally displaced fractures. For impacted fracture there will be distortion of normal bone architecture by compression of bone, but there has been no separation of the fracture surfaces (Fig. 2.3). A minimally displaced fracture is one where the fracture surfaces are just beginning to displace (Fig. 2.9). This is clearly an area of some confusion but inevitably there will be degrees of displacement. No clear cut-off point exists between displaced and undisplaced fractures. As a rough guide the fracture can still be classified as undisplaced provided there has been only a mild or moderate degree of displacement or angulation at the fracture site on either AP or lateral X-ray.

Further subdivision of intracapsular fractures is of doubtful value. Whilst a number of classification systems exist, they suffer from problems of interobserver variations and are of little more value in predicting healing complication than the simpler division into displaced and undisplaced fractures.

Alternative classification

The Garden grading (Fig. 2.10) is still quoted in many publications in the literature. This classification is based purely on the appearance of the femoral head on the AP X-ray. The four divisions are dependent on the displacement of the trabeculae within the femoral head from their normal alignment with those of the acetabulum and from their normal 160° angle with the femoral shaft. The classification

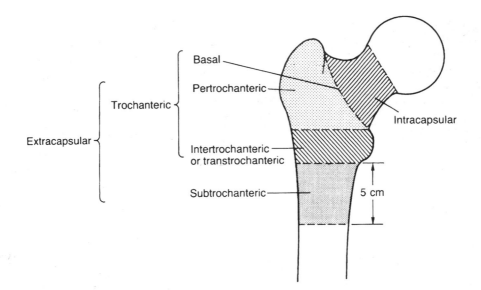

Fig. 2.7   Primary classification of proximal femoral fractures.

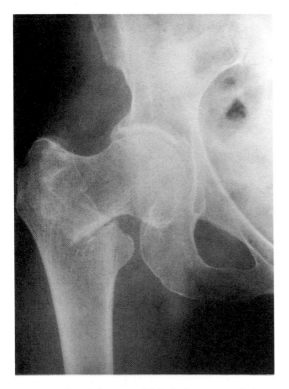

Fig. 2.8   A basal fracture. This is best regarded as an extracapsular fracture.

is not of better value than the division of fractures into undisplaced fractures (grade 1 and 2) and displaced fractures (grade 3 and 4):

1 *Garden 1.* There is impaction laterally in the femoral neck, which results in a more vertical position of the femoral head trabeculae (trabecular angle 165–180°). Alternative names which have been used for this fracture are impaction, abduction or valgus fractures.
2 *Garden 2.* There is no displacement of impaction of the fracture, therefore the trabeculae maintain their normal alignment (160°).
3 *Garden 3.* The proximal displacement of the distal fragment has allowed the femoral head to rotate to a more horizontal position by the cog-wheeling effect between the bone ends. The trabecular angle is less than 160°.
4 *Garden 4.* There is no contact between the fracture surfaces and cog-wheeling does not occur. The femoral head trabeculae resume their normal alignment with the acetabulum and femoral shaft.

Other methods of classification

The Pauwels classification is based on the angle of the fracture line with the horizontal but has little clinical relevance. The AO classification has nine subdivisions but is of doubtful practical value. The division into subcapital and cervical fractures is dependent

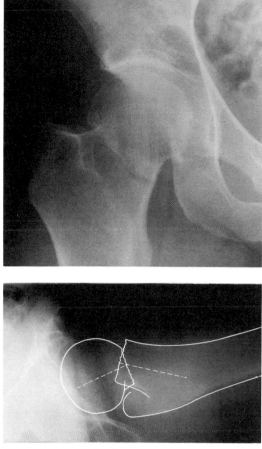

(a)

(b)

Fig. 2.9 An intracapsular fracture which is impacted on (a) the anteroposterior view. (b) On the lateral view there has been some impaction of the fracture surfaces with 40° of angulation between the fracture surfaces. Traditionally this fracture is still classified as an undisplaced fracture.

on the distance of the fracture from the joint line, with subcapital fractures being more proximal. Whilst this may have a slight difference on outcome, it is insufficient to justify the distinction. Other terms used in the classification of intracapsular fractures are medial femoral neck fractures, adduction, impacted, valgus, varus, transcervical, mid cervical and basicervical. To avoid confusion these terms are best avoided.

Classification of extracapsular fractures

Extracapsular fractures are subdivided into trochanteric and subtrochanteric fractures

(Fig. 2.7). Even this simple separation can cause confusion, particularly if the fracture line crosses these anatomical boundaries. The actual level at which trochanteric and subtrochanteric fractures are divided is also debatable. Traditional classifications, such as those proposed by Fielding and Magliato (1966); Zickel (1976) and Seinsheimer (1978), included fractures at the level of the lesser trochanter with subtrochanteric fractures. The more recent AO classification includes only those distal to the lower part of the lesser trochanter.

The dividing point between a subtrochanteric fracture and a femoral diaphyseal fracture is also open to question. Most papers recommend a distance of 5 cm from the distal

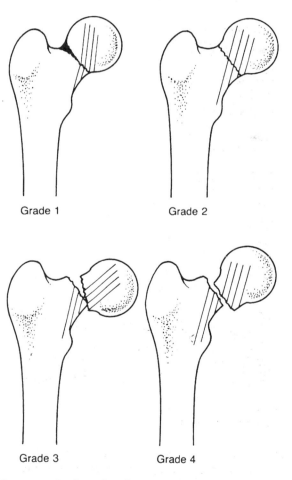

Grade 1 Grade 2

Grade 3 Grade 4

Fig. 2.10 Garden classification of intracapsular fractures.

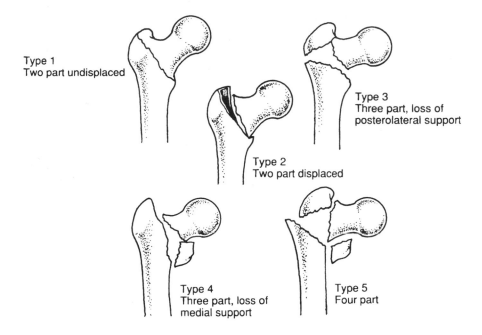

Type 1
Two part undisplaced

Type 3
Three part, loss of
posterolateral support

Type 2
Two part displaced

Type 4
Three part, loss of
medial support

Type 5
Four part

Fig. 2.11   Jensen classification of trochanteric fractures.

part of the lesser trochanter, although the AO classification suggests a distance of 3 cm.

Many different classification systems have been proposed for extracapsular fractures. The most important are presented here:

- Evans in 1949 described one of the first classification systems of trochanteric fractures, depending on the appearance of the fracture following reduction.
- Jensen and Michaelsen (1975) modified the Evans classification to subclassify only those fractures which traversed the femur between the lesser and greater trochanter into five groups (Fig. 2.11).
- Fielding and Magliato (1966) described a simple subdivision of subtrochanteric fractures (Fig. 2.12). The type chosen depended on the level at which the fracture line was predominantly located.
- Seinsheimer (1978) described a widely used classification of subtrochanteric fractures (Fig. 2.13). It included any femur fracture in which any part of the fracture line was within the 5 cm of bone distal to the lesser trochanter.
- AO classification of fractures divides trochanteric fractures into nine groups and

subtrochanteric into six groups (Fig. 2.14). Subtrochanteric fractures are defined as those in which the fracture line traverses the femur in the 3 cm distal to the lesser trochanter.

- Zickel (1976) subdivided subtrochanteric fractures into six groups, which included fractures within the proximal third of the femoral diaphysis.

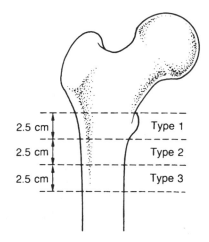

2.5 cm   Type 1

2.5 cm   Type 2

2.5 cm   Type 3

Fig. 2.12   Fielding classification of subtrochanteric fractures.

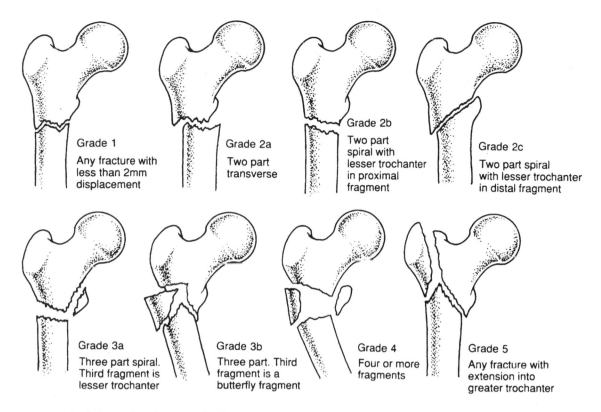

Fig. 2.13 Seinsheimer classification of subtrochanteric fractures.

To avoid confusion, until a universal classification system is developed, the following guidelines on fracture classification are recommended for extracapsular fractures.

1 The level of the fracture is determined by the region of the femur in which the fracture line traversing the femur is predominantly present.
2 'True' subtrochanteric fractures are those found from a transverse line at the distal margin of the lesser trochanter to 5 cm distal to this.
3 Basal fractures are two-part fractures in which the fracture plane runs along the line of capsular insertion, just proximal to the lesser and greater trochanter. They are best considered as trochanteric fractures.
4 A number of different terms have been used for trochanteric fractures. 'Pertrochanteric' (through) refers to a fracture running obliquely between the greater and lesser trochanter. The term 'intertrochanteric' (between) traditionally refers to a more transverse fracture line running from below the greater trochanter to above the lesser trochanter. However many surgeons use these terms interchangeably. The term transtrochanteric fracture refers to a fracture line at the level of the lesser trochanter. All these terms can cause confusion and it is therefore recommended to use only the term 'trochanteric'.
5 Trochanteric fracture may be subdivided by the Jensen classification (Fig. 2.11), with type 1 and 2 fracture being regarded as 'stable' and types 3, 4 and 5 as comminuted or 'unstable'.
6 Subtrochanteric fractures are infrequent and can simply be subdivided into undisplaced, two-part and comminuted fractures.

Figure 2.15 summarizes the classification of hip fractures.

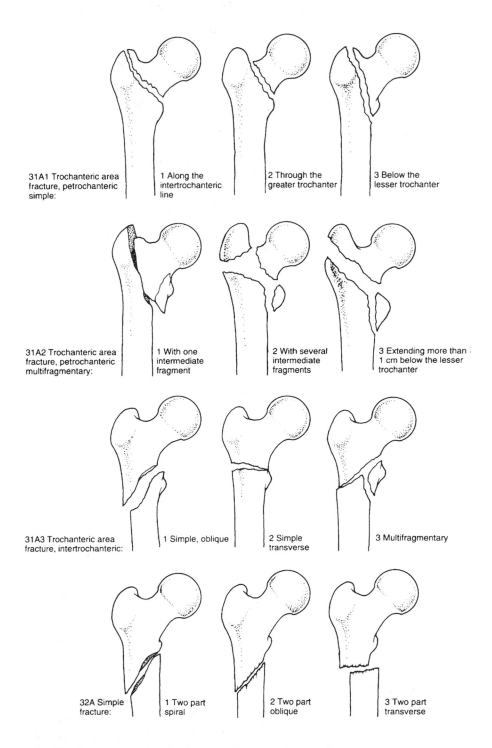

31A1 Trochanteric area fracture, petrochanteric simple:	1 Along the intertrochanteric line	2 Through the greater trochanter	3 Below the lesser trochanter
31A2 Trochanteric area fracture, petrochanteric multifragmentary:	1 With one intermediate fragment	2 With several intermediate fragments	3 Extending more than 1 cm below the lesser trochanter
31A3 Trochanteric area fracture, intertrochanteric:	1 Simple, oblique	2 Simple transverse	3 Multifragmentary
32A Simple fracture:	1 Two part spiral	2 Two part oblique	3 Two part transverse

Fig. 2.14   AO classification of extracapsular fractures.

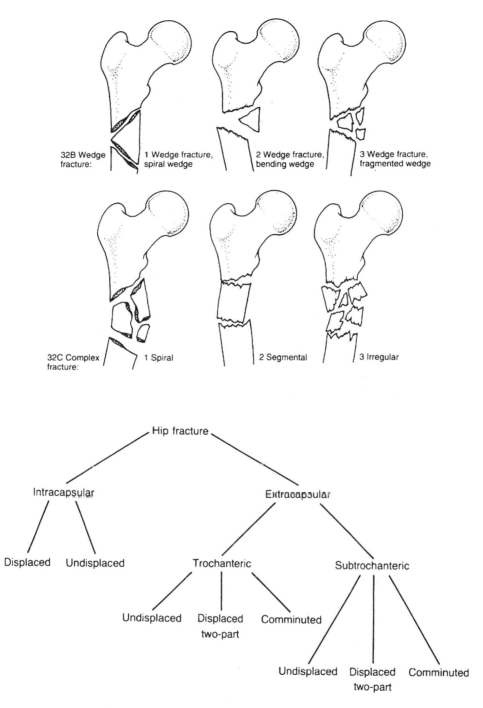

Fig. 2.15 Classification of hip fractures.

Treatment options

It is not possible to specify exactly which type of treatment should be used for each type of fracture. Many factors need to be considered, other than the type of fracture (Table 2.1; Fig. 2.16). Surgical treatment is inappropriate if there is not access to a fully equipped orthopaedic theatre with an appropriately trained surgeon and supporting staff. The presence of

Table 2.1 Factors which need to be considered in determining the choice of treatment

Associated injuries
Other medical conditions
Age of the patient
Rheumatoid arthritis
Presence of Paget's disease
Is the fracture secondary to malignancy?
Presence of metabolic bone disease
Resources available for treatment
Patient preferences

other injuries or medical conditions may take preference over treatment of the hip fracture. Other specific medical conditions may also dictate the choice of treatment. This will be discussed further in later chapters.

Conservative treatment of undisplaced intracapsular fractures

Currently the majority of orthopaedic surgeons recommend that undisplaced intracapsular fractures should be treated operatively by internal fixation, to reduce the risk of the fracture becoming displaced. The difference between operative and conservative treatment can be summarized as follows:

1 Operative treatment will reduce the risk of non-union/early displacement of the fracture from approximately 15% to 5%. Most fractures that displace will require arthroplasty, as opposed to the more minor operation of internal fixation.
2 Operative treatment allows aspiration of any haematoma from within the hip joint. This may reduce the risk of avascular necrosis developing later.
3 Operative treatment enables the patient to be mobilized with greater confidence. The length of hospital stay and the need for follow-up may therefore be reduced.
4 Conservative treatment will reduce the overall number of patients requiring surgical treatment. If routine internal fixation

is performed then approximately 95% of patients will require one operation and 5% two operations. With conservative treatment only approximately 15% will require surgery.

If conservative treatment is planned it should be reserved for those intracapsular fractures that show impaction. The exact treatment regime varies between different centres which practise conservative treatment. Some recommend a period of a few days' bed rest prior to mobilization with partial weight-bearing. Others advocate immediate mobilization with no restriction on weight-bearing. Regular radiographic follow-up is however required, with surgical intervention should the fracture show signs of displacement.

Internal fixation of intracapsular fractures

The following types of intracapsular fractures may be treated by internal fixation.

Indications for internal fixation of intracapsular fractures

Undisplaced intracapsular fractures

Minimally displaced intracapsular fractures

Displaced intracapsular fractures in the 'young'

Displaced intracapsular fractures in the 'elderly' (see discussion)

Undisplaced intracapsular fractures

These fractures may be treated by internal fixation or managed conservatively. Arthroplasty which has greater morbidity is inappropriate for this type of fracture.

Minimally displaced intracapsular fractures

Approximately 10% of intracapsular fractures will be essentially undisplaced on one radiographic projection, yet moderately displaced on the other view. Opinion differs between orthopaedic surgeons as to whether these

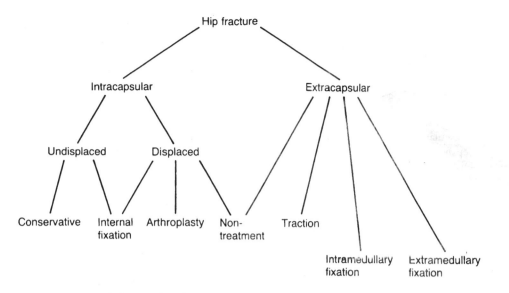

Fig. 2.16   Treatment options following hip fracture.

should be classified as displaced or undisplaced fractures. It is however recommended that these fractures be treated by internal fixation as this is the simpler procedure. The incidence of non-union or early displacement of the fracture is comparable to that for an undisplaced intracapsular fracture.

Displaced intracapsular fractures in the young

For those patients whose life expectancy is more than 5–8 years, preservation of the femoral head is desirable. This is because a successfully united femoral head is less likely to cause long-term complications than that of even the most effective hip arthroplasty. In addition, revision surgery following internal fixation is much simpler than that following a hip arthroplasty.

Opinions differ as to what constitutes a 'young' patient. An arbitrary age limit of 70 years of age is frequently quoted, although it is preferable to consider a physiological age. Using such an assessment, a young patient is one who is physically active and able to walk distances in excess of 800 metres with minimal use of walking aids. Such patients have a low mortality following a hip fracture, and if an arthroplasty is performed have a significant risk of developing long-term complications

related to the prosthesis. Reduction and internal fixation are therefore recommended for these patients.

Displaced intracapsular fractures in the elderly

This is an area of considerable controversy as to the preferred method of treatment. This type of fracture has frequently been termed the unsolved fracture. Both internal fixation and arthroplasty have their own advantages and disadvantages. These are summarized in Table 2.2.

Non-union
This is the main concern with internal fixation. Incidence rates quoted vary considerably and are highly influenced by factors. For displaced intracapsular fractures in the elderly an incidence of approximately 20–30% should be expected. Arthroplasty therefore avoids this complication.

Avascular necrosis
An incidence of approximately 10–20% can be expected following internal fixation. However in many of these cases symptoms are minimal and revision surgery is only required in a small proportion of cases.

Sepsis around implant
Whilst infrequent, this is a devastating complication with a mortality in excess of 50%. It

Table 2.2 Differences between internal fixation and arthroplasty (see text for clarification)

	Internal fixation	Arthroplasty
Non-union	Incurred	Avoided
Avascular necrosis	Incurred	Avoided
Sepsis around implant	Rare	Occasional
Dislocation	Avoided	Occasional
Acetabular erosion	Avoided	Rare
Prosthesis loosening	Avoided	Occasional
Re-fracture around implant	Rare	Occasional
Re-operation rate	High	Fairly low
Mortality	May be reduced	May be increased
Hospital stay	May be reduced	May be increased
Cost of treatment	May be reduced	May be increased

is a rare complication following internal fixation, especially if a percutaneous surgical technique is used. Following arthroplasty an incidence of approximately 2–5% can be expected.

Dislocation
This complication is only incurred after arthroplasty. For a hemiarthroplasty an incidence of approximately 4% can be expected. If a total hip replacement is used the incidence is increased to approximately 10%. Dislocation represents a major complication in the frail elderly, with approximately 50% of patients dying soon afterwards.

Acetabular erosion
This complication only occurs after hemiarthroplasty. An overall incidence of 20% can be expected in long-term survivors. Few patients will require revision surgery for this, especially amongst the elderly population.

Prosthesis loosening
This also only occurs after arthroplasty, with an incidence of approximately 10%. The incidence can be reduced by cementing the prosthesis. Not all cases of loosening will however require revision surgery.

Re-fracture around implant
This refers to a second fracture which occurs around or more commonly just below the prosthesis. It is an unusual complication following internal fixation and tends to be specific to certain types of implants. It is more frequent following an arthroplasty, with an incidence of 2–4%. Treatment of this complication is demanding, with a high mortality and morbidity in the elderly.

Re-operation rate
Following internal fixation a re-operation rate of up to 25–30% can be expected. Two-thirds of these operations will be conversion to an arthroplasty for non-union of the fracture. Implant removal because of discomfort will account for approximately one-sixth of the re-operations and the remainder will be for a variety of indications such as avascular necrosis.

A re-operation rate of approximately 10% can be expected after arthroplasty. Operations required will be for reduction of dislocation, drainage of sepsis or fixation of fractures around the implant. All these re-operations are associated with a high mortality.

Mortality
Many individual studies have failed to find any difference in mortality between internal fixation or arthroplasty, but meta-analysis of all the studies suggests that early mortality is reduced following internal fixation.

Hospital stay and cost of treatment

Internal fixation is probably, associated with a reduced hospital stay and this results in a slightly reduced cost of treatment.

There have been a number of randomized trials comparing outcome for displaced intracapsular fractures in the elderly treated by internal fixation or arthroplasty. Results of studies to date have been conflicting. At present it is not possible to state confidently which is the best method of treatment for this type of fracture. Treatment will therefore be dictated by the available facilities and particular expertise of each individual surgeon. Currently Scandinavian countries tend to favour internal fixation, whilst in much of Europe and the USA arthroplasty is preferred.

Arthroplasty

The following types of intracapsular fractures may be treated with an arthroplasty.

Indications for arthroplasty in the treatment of a proximal femoral fracture

Displaced intracapsular fractures with a significant delay in diagnosis

Displaced intracapsular fractures in patients with rheumatoid arthritis

Intracapsular fractures secondary to Paget's disease

Intracapsular fractures secondary to malignancy

Intracapsular fractures associated with metabolic bone disease

Hip fracture with coexistent arthritis of the hip

Displaced intracapsular fractures in the elderly (see discussion)

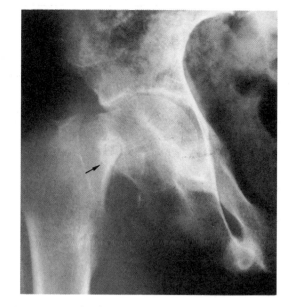

Fig. 2.17 A displaced intracapsular fracture in which the diagnosis was delayed. There is an area of dense bone where the fracture surface have impacted (arrow), with a distinct line at the fracture surface where the bone ends have been articulating together.

Displaced intracapsular fractures in the elderly

The arguments for and against this method of treatment, in comparison with internal fixation, have already been discussed.

Displaced intracapsular fractures with a delay in diagnosis

The fracture may show the characteristic features illustrated in Fig. 2.17. Because impaction has occurred at the fracture site it will be impossible to reduce such a fracture with a closed reduction.

Clinical studies indicate that from 1 week after the time of fracture the incidence of non-union will increase considerably. In this situation arthroplasty is preferable in all but very young patients, where open reduction and a revascularization procedure may be more appropriate.

For the time period up to 1 week from injury, the larger studies which have considered this question found no significant increase in the incidence of non-union. There have however been a few studies which have suggested that non-union is more common if surgery is delayed by only a few hours. This is an area of continuing controversy.

Intracapsular fractures in patients with rheumatoid arthritis

For patients who have rheumatoid arthritis with an undisplaced intracapsular fracture, internal fixation is probably not associated with any increase in the risk of healing complications. For displaced intracapsular fractures treated by reduction and internal fixation, over half will develop non-union; furthermore, avascular necrosis is more frequent. This has led to the recommendation that displaced intracapsular fractures in patients with rheumatoid arthritis should always be treated by replacement arthroplasty.

Intracapsular fractures secondary to Paget's disease

Clinical studies have indicated that internal fixation of intracapsular fractures caused by Paget's disease consistently results in non-union. Arthroplasty is therefore indicated for this type of fracture. There is insufficient evidence within the literature to be able to give treatment guidelines for undisplaced intracapsular fractures with Paget's.

Intracapsular fractures secondary to malignancy

Internal fixation of pathological intracapsular fractures is not recommended as it invariably leads to non-union, with a painful functionless hip. Arthroplasty is therefore indicated.

Intracapsular fractures in the presence of metabolic bone disease

Chronic renal failure and hyperparathyroidism result in an increased risk of fracture non-union. Reports in the literature state that non-union occurs in all intracapsular fractures treated by internal fixation, regardless of the degree of displacement. Arthroplasty is therefore indicated if chronic renal failure is present.

Table 2.3   Implants that have been used for extramedullary fixation of extracapsular fractures

Static extramedullary implants	Dynamic extramedullary implants
Thornton nail plate	Dynamic hip screw
McLaughlin nail plate	Richards hip screw
Jewett nail plate	Massie nail
95° AO blade plate	Pugh nail
95° Dynamic compression screw	Ambi hip screw
	Medoff sliding plate

Hip fracture with coexistent arthritis (arthrosis) of the hip

Arthritis of the hip reduces the risk of sustaining an intracapsular fracture, but has no effect on the risk of extracapsular fracture. If the degree of arthritis of the hip is significant total hip replacement is the choice of treatment.

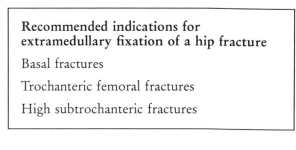

> **Recommended indications for extramedullary fixation of a hip fracture**
>
> Basal fractures
>
> Trochanteric femoral fractures
>
> High subtrochanteric fractures

Extramedullary fixation of extracapsular fractures

This refers to implants which have a pin or screw connected to a plate on the lateral side of the femur. These implants can be divided into static and dynamic implants. Table 2.3 lists the implants that have been most frequently used.

The static implants (Fig. 2.18) have a solid single nail attached to the side plate. These implants have problems with cutting out of the femoral head and penetration into the hip joint, as the fracture collapses. In addition they are mechanically weaker with a greater risk of breaking than the newer dynamic implants. Numerous studies have shown them

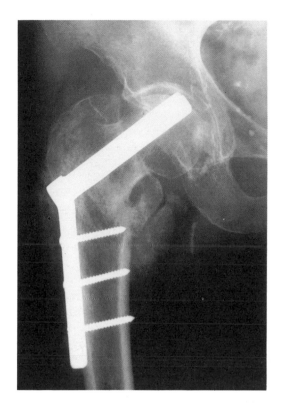

Fig. 2.18 A fixed or static nail plate in which there is no capacity for sliding of the cross pin as the fracture collapses. This results in an unacceptably high risk of penetration of the implant into the hip joint, as illustrated here.

to be inferior to dynamic implants and therefore their use can no longer be justified.

Dynamic implants, of which the dynamic hip screw (DHS) is the most prevalent, are now the choice of implant for the majority of extracapsular femoral fractures. The term Dynamic Hip Screw is synonymous with the term compression hip screw, sliding hip screw and equivalent models such as the Richards or Ambi hip screws. They are designed to allow limited collapse at the fracture site as the bone heals. Numerous studies have shown this type of implant to have a lower incidence of healing complications in comparison to both static nail plates and Ender's intramedullary nails.

The gamma nail is a recently introduced intramedullary implant for the treatment of extracapsular fractures. It has been well-evaluated in a number of randomized trials comparing it with the DHS; results indicate

that, whilst the two implants have a similar cut-out rate, the gamma nail has a significantly increased re-operation rate. This is due to a risk of fracture around the nail, both during surgery and in the postoperative period. The insertion of the gamma nail is also somewhat more demanding for the surgeon to perform. These complications preclude the routine use of this implant; nevertheless a longer version of the original gamma nail may be of value for subtrochanteric fractures as there have been encouraging preliminary reports of its use.

Subtrochanteric fractures have a considerably higher incidence of fracture-healing complications in comparison to trochanteric fractures. This is due to the high mechanical forces acting in this area (Fig. 2.19).

Much of the problem with DHS fixation of a subtrochanteric fracture is that, as the fracture line becomes more distal, the DHS stops performing as a dynamic implant and acts as a static implant (Fig. 2.20). This leads to the associated complications of static fixation, such as delayed fracture healing, non-union, plate breakage and cut-out. These problems have led many surgeons to treat these fractures with an intramedullary implant. There

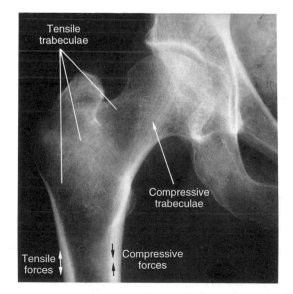

Fig. 2.19 The subtrochanteric area has compressive forces on the medial femoral cortex and tensile forces on the lateral cortex.

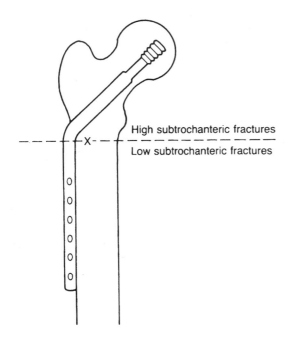

High subtrochanteric fractures

Low subtrochanteric fractures

Fig. 2.20 As the fracture line becomes more distal, the bone in area X on the proximal side of the fracture stops the sliding of the dynamic hip screw (DHS) and forces it to act as a static implant. For a high subtrochanteric fracture the fracture line is at the level of the lower border of the lesser trochanter and the DHS can still act as a dynamic implant.

are however few comparative studies to compare intramedullary with extramedullary implants for this type of fracture to allow firm treatment guidelines to be made.

Intramedullary fixation of extracapsular fractures

> **Recommended indications for intramedullary fixation of a hip fracture**
>
> Low subtrochanteric fractures
>
> Hip fracture with associated femoral shaft fracture
>
> Pathological extracapsular fractures

This refers to the insertion of a nail via the greater trochanter into the intramedullary canal of the femur. Cross screws are passed through the nail into the femoral head and neck. Examples of these implants include gamma nail, Küntscher-Y nail, Richards intramedullary hip screw, Richards reconstruction nail, Variwall reconstruction nail and Zickel nail. Enders nails are an exception to this; they are flexible metal rods which are passed up the femoral shaft from the femoral condyles. However they have a significant increased risk of fixation failure which precludes their routine use.

For low subtrochanteric fractures (Fig. 2.21) an intramedullary implant is probably the treatment of choice. Early results of comparative studies of a gamma nail with the DHS for subtrochanteric fractures have indicated reduced operation times and blood loss for the gamma nail. The use of intramedullary nails is discussed in Chapter 7.

Rarely a hip fracture is associated with a fracture of the femoral shaft (Fig. 2.22). In this situation optimal fixation may be with an intramedullary nail to stabilize both fractures.

Pathological extracapsular fractures with extensive tumour in the proximal femur are probably better treated with an intramedullary nail (Fig. 2.23), as DHS fixation has a risk of fracture occurring below the plate (Fig. 2.24).

Traction for extracapsular hip fractures

> **Indications for treating extracapsular fractures by traction**
>
> Patient refuses to consent to surgery
>
> Patient unfit for any form of anaesthesia
>
> Lack of modern surgical facilities
>
> Lack of appropriately trained surgeon

Treatment of an intracapsular fracture by traction is not appropriate. Extracapsular fractures have historically been treated using traction with reasonable results. Hornby and colleagues (1989), in a randomized trial, compared traction with operative treatment. They

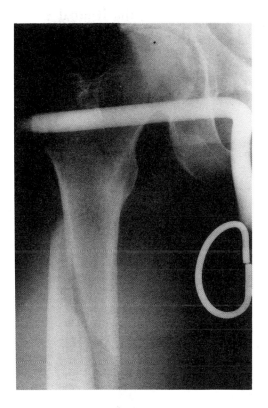

Fig. 2.21 A spiral subtrochanteric fracture. Such a fracture may be fixed with a Dynamic Hip Screw but this would require a long side plate with extensive surgical exposure. Furthermore the DHS will be acting as a 'static' implant. Fixation with an intramedullary nail is therefore probably more appropriate.

found similar mortality for both treatments, but a greatly increased proportion of patients who had a prolonged hospital stay (and presumably loss of independence), following treatment with traction. Treatment of extracapsular fractures by traction should therefore be reserved for those indications listed above. The technical details of how to apply traction and aftercare are beyond the scope of this book.

Non-treatment

There will be a very small group of patients presenting with a hip fracture in whom specific treatment of the fracture is not appropriate. Non-treatment needs to be clearly

distinguished from conservative treatment. For conservative treatment specific measures are taken to ensure that the fracture heals in good alignment, enabling return of hip function.

Non-treatment should be reserved for a small selected group of patients. For those in whom survival is expected to be less than a few weeks, surgery is inappropriate. In addition there will be a small group of patients who are totally immobile before the fracture, in whom the benefits of surgery are debatable. Whilst surgery in such patients will not restore mobility, it does make the management of such a patient easier, as the injured limb can still be used for standing, when

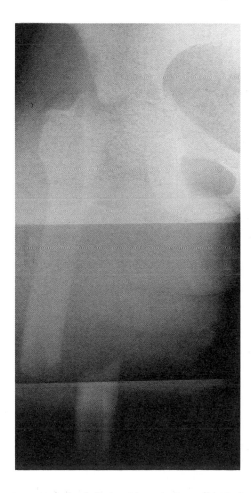

Fig. 2.22 Femoral shaft and neck fracture. Each fracture may be stabilized separately, or alternatively one implant may be used for both fractures.

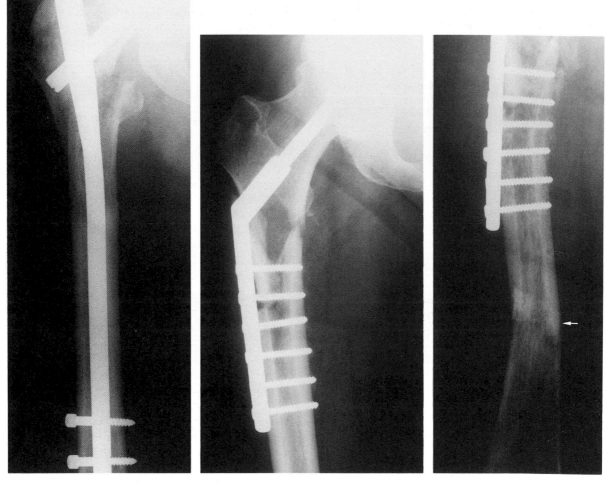

Fig. 2.23 Pathological fracture at the level of the lesser trochanter with tumour destroying the femur distal to the lesser trochanter. The fracture was treated with a long gamma nail.

Fig. 2.24 A subtrochanteric fracture caused by metastasis from carcinoma of the breast. Whilst the initial postoperative X-ray may appear adequate, because of the extensive tumour within the femur a fracture distal to the plate (arrow) occurred 3 months later.

moving the patient from bed to chair. Furthermore, pain in the injured hip is less of a problem following surgery.

Non-treatment involves resting the limb in the position of comfort, skilled nursing care to avoid pressure sores, and analgesia as appropriate. It is frequently found that strong analgesics such as opiates will be needed for some weeks from injury. As soon as pain permits, the patient may be allowed to sit and later to stand as able. For intracapsular fractures non-union invariably occurs with the hip functioning similar to after a Girdlestone-type procedure. For extracapsular fracture there may eventually be fracture union in some cases, albeit with a shortening and external rotation deformity.

In conclusion, non-treatment should be reserved for a small and carefully selected group of patients. Skilled nursing care is a prerequisite and will invariably be required for the rest of the patient's life. Strong analgesia may be required for some weeks after injury.

Key references on diagnosis

Egund N, Nilsson LT, Wingstrand H, Strömqvist B, Pettersson H. CT scans and lipohaemarthrosis in hip fractures. *J Bone Joint Surg* 1990; **72–B**:379–382.

Evans PD, Wilson C, Lyons K. Comparison of MRI with bone scanning for suspected hip fracture in elderly patients. *J Bone Joint Surg* 1994; **76–B**:158–159.

Holder LE, Schwarz C, Wernicke PG, Michael RH. Radionuclide bone imaging in the early detection of fractures of the proximal femur (hip): multifactorial analysis. *Radiology* 1990; **174**:509–515.

O'Dwyer FG, Harper WM, Finlay DB. Do elderly patients with hip pain following trauma require hospital admission? *Injury* 1992; **23**:295–296.

Rizzo PF, Gould ES, Lyden JP, Asnis SE. Diagnosis of occult fractures about the hip; magnetic resonance imaging compared with bone-scanning. *J Bone Joint Surg* 1993; **75–A**:395–401.

Key references on fracture classification

Editorial. Reporting hip fractures in the elderly. *Acta Orthop Scand* 1988; **59**:359–360.

Eliasson P, Hansson LI, Kärrholm J. Displacement in femoral neck fractures: a numerical analysis of 200 fractures. *Acta Orthop Scand* 1988; **59**:361–364.

Evans EM. The treatment of trochanteric fractures of the femur. *J Bone Joint Surg* 1949; **31–B**:190–203.

Fielding JW, Magliato HJ. Subtrochanteric fractures. *Surg Gynecol Obstet* 1966; **122**:555–560.

Garden RS. Low-angle fixation in fractures of the femoral neck. *J Bone Joint Surg* 1961; **43–B**:647–663.

Jensen JS, Michaelsen M. Trochanteric femoral fractures treated with McLaughlin osteosynthesis. *Acta Orthop Scand* 1975; **46**:795–803.

Müller ME, Nazarian S, Koch P, Schatzker J. *The AO Classification of Fracture of Long Bones*. Springer-Verlag, Berlin, 1990.

Parker MJ, Pryor GA. *Hip Fracture Management*. Blackwell Scientific Publications, Oxford, 1993.

Seinsheimer F. Subtrochanteric fractures of the femur. *J Bone Joint Surg* 1978; **60–A**:300–306.

Zickel RE. An intramedullary fixation device for the proximal part of the femur. *J Bone Joint Surg* 1976; **58–A**:866–872.

Key references on treatment options

Barnes R, Brown JT, Garden RS, Nicoll EA. Subcapital fractures of the femur: a prospective review. *J Bone Joint Surg* 1976; **58–B**:2–24.

Bogoch E, Ouellette G, Hastings D. Failure of internal fixation of displaced femoral neck fractures in rheumatoid patients. *J Bone Joint Surg* 1991; **73–B**:7–10.

Dove J. Complete fractures of the femur in Paget's disease of bone. *J Bone Joint Surg* 1980; **62–B**:12–17.

Galasko CSB. The management of skeletal metastases. *J R Coll Surg Edinb* 1980; **25**:143–161.

Hornby R, Grimley Evans J, Vardon V. Operative or conservative treatment for trochanteric fractures of the femur: a randomised epidemiological trial in elderly patients. *J Bone Joint Surg* 1989; **71–B**:619–623.

Jensen JS, Sonne-Holm S, Tøndevold E. Unstable trochanteric fractures: a comparative analysis of four methods of internal fixation. *Acta Orthop Scand* 1980; **51**:949–962.

Lu-yao GL, Keller RB, Littenberg B, Wennberg JE. Outcomes after displaced fractures of the femoral neck: a meta-analysis of one hundred and six published reports. *J Bone Joint Surg* 1994; **76–A**:15–25.

Parker MJ. Internal fixation or arthroplasty for displaced subcapital fractures in the elderly. *Injury* 1992; **23**:521–524.

Parker MJ, Pryor GA. Gamma verses DHS nailing for extracapsular femoral fractures: meta-analysis of ten randomised trails. *Int Orthop* 1996; **20**:163–168.

Parker MJ, Robinson CM. Gamma nail versus sliding hip screw for the treatment of extracapsular fracture of the proximal femur. In: Gillespie WJ, Madhok R, Swiontkowski M, Robinson CM, Murray GD (eds.) Musculoskeletal injuries Module of The Cochrane Database of Systematic Reviews. Available in The Cochrane Library [database on disk and CDROM]. The Cochrane Collaboration; Oxford: Update software: 1996. BMJ publishing group, London.

Raaymakers ELFB, Marti RK. Non-operative treatment of impacted femoral neck fractures: a prospective study of 170 cases. *J Bone Joint Surg* 1991; **73–B**:950–954.

Strömqvist B, Nilsson LT, Thorngren K-G. Femoral neck fracture fixation with hook-pins: 2-year results and learning curve in 626 prospective cases. *Acta Orthop Scand* 1992; **63**:282–287.

Swiontkowski MF. Intracapsular fractures of the hip. *J Bone Joint Surg* 1994; **76–A**:129–138.

3

Patient assessment and initial management

Medical assessment

The average age of a patient presenting with a hip fracture will be around 80 years but their physical and mental well-being is likely to be inferior to the average 80-year-old. Multiple medical problems are often present, making full assessment on admission essential. Moreover, as most will require surgery it is important that the medical state of these patients is optimum at the time of surgery and remains so afterwards.

Particular areas requiring special consideration in hip fracture patients are as follows:

Injuries sustained from the fall

Is the hip fracture an isolated fracture or are there other injuries? A fractured wrist or neck of humerus is the commonest associated injury.

Cardiac function

Evidence of impaired cardiac function is frequently found in hip fracture patients. This can generally be adequately assessed for most patients from the clinical history and examination supplemented by an electrocardiogram (ECG) and chest X-ray. Uncontrolled cardiac failure, significant arrhythmias or hypertension should be treated prior to surgery.

Respiratory function

Deterioration in respiratory function may occur between sustaining the fracture and surgery due to immobility, or rarely fat embolism. The aim should be to achieve optimum respiratory function prior to surgery.

Renal function

This should be checked preoperatively. If the urea or creatinine is elevated the cause should be investigated. It is most commonly secondary to prerenal failure from dehydration. Ideally the urea should not be above 10 mmol/l at the time of surgery. A urine sample should be obtained and tested for sugar, protein and infection.

Neurological function

Impairment of neurological or locomotive function may be implicated in the aetiology of the fall and may occasionally be improved by appropriate treatment.

Parkinson's disease

This is frequently implicated in the aetiology of the fall. The diagnosis may need to be considered in those with clinical features suggestive of the disease, that is tremor, akinesia and rigidity. The hospital stay for the hip fracture be may be used to adjust or initiate appropriate therapy.

Visual deficiency

Poor vision is one of the aetiological factors for hip fracture. Treatable causes should be sought.

Previous stroke

Patients who have had a stroke are more likely to sustain a hip fracture and the fracture tends to be on the paralysed side.

Thyroid function

Hyperthyroidism or excessive thyroxine medication results in osteoporosis. Hypothyroidism may be implicated in the aetiology of the fall.

Pre-fracture mobility

An accurate record of the pre-fracture mobility should be made, using such questions as total walking distance, ability to do shopping and use of walking aids. Comparison can then be made to this over the recovery period. Furthermore the pre-fracture mobility is one of the most significant predictors of mortality and morbidity following a hip fracture. A further prediction of outcome is the ability of the patient to visit friends, as this represents a combined indicator of physical and mental fitness.

Activities of daily living

A record of the patient's capabilities prior to the fracture should be made. This should

Table 3.1 Abbreviated mental test score

State age
Give current time to the nearest hour
When given an address to remember, repeat it at the end of the test (e.g. 42 Alexandria Road, Birmingham)
State present year
Give the name of the institution to which you have been admitted
Recognize two persons (e.g. nurse, doctor)
State date of birth (day and month are sufficient)
Give the year of the start of the Second World War
Give the name of the present monarch or head of state
Count backwards from 20 to 1

include the patient's ability to carry out household functions, bathing, toilet and capability to climb stairs. Each function can be recorded separately or alternatively, combined to form an overall score such as the Barthel index.

Social function

Many patients who come from their own home may have difficulty coping at home or will be dependent on others. Subsequent planning of discharge will need to be made with the full knowledge of the patient's capabilities prior to the injury.

Mental state

Pre-fracture mental state is a useful predictor of mortality and morbidity following a hip fracture. A standard method of assessment is the 10-point mental state score (Table 3.1). A low score is not diagnostic of dementia, but may be due to other causes such as an acute confusion state.

Table 3.2 Drugs that have been implicated in the aetiology of hip fractures

Increased incidence	Reduced incidence
Steroids	Hormone replacement therapy
Sedatives	Thiazide diuretics
Anticonvulsants	Calcium
Thyroxine	Vitamin D
	Diphosphonates

Bone strength

As discussed in Chapter 1, there are a number of conditions which result in reduced bone strength. Treatment of these conditions may be merited.

Medication

The hospital stay for a hip fracture should be used as an opportunity for the rationalization of any drug therapy. In addition the long-term use of any drug that may be implicated in the aetiology of the hip fracture should be reviewed (Table 3.2).

Drug allergies

Prophylactic antibiotics should be used in the perioperative period. A history of drug allergies should be considered when making the choice.

Previous thrombotic or haemorrhagic events

A history of previous thrombosis will indicate that more intensive thrombotic-preventive measures should be considered. A history of recent or recurrent haemorrhagic events will be a contraindication to pharmacological prophylaxis.

Anaemia

The haemoglobin needs to be checked to obtain a baseline and if anaemia is present it may require further investigation. A rough guide is that surgery should be delayed until the haemoglobin is 100 g/l, or above.

Nutrition

Many hip fracture patients have an inadequate dietary intake. The serum albumin and skin-fold thickness can be used to quantify the extent of malnutrition. Malnutrition will impair recovery and increase the risk of post-operative complications, and should be treated with appropriate nutrition supplements.

Paget's disease

One of the effects of this condition is weakening of the bone structure leading to pathological fractures. Other signs of the condition may also be present.

Malignant disease

Overt or occult malignant disease may be present in the elderly population of hip fracture patients. In addition the fracture may be caused by spread of malignant disease to the skeletal system. Clinical examination should therefore be comprehensive at the time of admission to hospital.

Potential sites of sepsis

Infection following surgery is a major complication. The presence of skin ulcers, cellulitis or other potential sites of sepsis should be sought. Acute infection, if present, should be corrected prior to surgery. Chronic leg ulcers should not be considered as an absolute contraindication to surgery, but in these patients the use of long-term prophylactic antibiotics should be considered.

Table 3.3 American Society of Anesthesiologists classification of physical status

Grade	Description
ASA 1	Completely fit and healthy
ASA 2	Some illness, but this has no effect on normal daily activity, that is, an asymptomatic condition such as hypertension
ASA 3	Symptomatic illness present, but minimal restriction on life, e.g. mild diabetes mellitus
ASA 4	Symptomatic illness causing severe restriction, e.g. severe chronic bronchitis, unstable diabetes
ASA 5	Moribund

Recurrent falls

The cause of the fall should be investigated to determine if there is a correctable cause, to reduce the chance of further injury.

Previous fractures

The history of previous fractures after minimal trauma indicates that preventive measures against further fractures should be considered.

Rheumatoid arthritis

The presence of clinical signs of this disease may indicate the choice of treatment with a tendency towards replacement arthroplasty. A lateral radiograph of the cervical spine should be taken in rheumatoid patients to exclude an instability within the cervical spine prior to administering general anaesthesia.

Overall physical state

A simple classification of the overall physical health of the patient can be made using the American Society of Anesthesiologists (ASA)

grade (Table 3.3). This has been shown to be predictive of mortality following hip fracture.

Preparation of the patient for theatre

As the majority of patients will be treated surgically, it is essential to ensure that the patient is presented for surgery as fit as possible. In addition appropriate prophylactic measures should be taken to prevent postoperative complications.

Routine preoperative investigations

The investigations shown below are routinely indicated following a hip fracture.

Routine investigations after hip fracture

Full blood count

Urea, glucose and electrolytes

Blood for cross-match, or group and save

Electrocardiogram

Chest X-ray

Urine analysis for protein and culture

Lateral cervical spine (patients with rheumatoid arthritis only)

Analgesia

The provision of adequate analgesia following a hip fracture is frequently neglected. The choice of analgesic is controversial. Available drugs are:

- *Aspirin or paracetamol*: These medications are of insufficient strength for an acute hip fracture but are of great value in the postoperative period. The same applies for compound preparations of aspirin or paracetamol.
- *Dihydrocodeine*: This is a stronger analgesic but has a strongly constipating effect,

especially in the immobile elderly patient.

- *Opiates*: These drugs form the mainstay of pain treatment for an acute hip fracture and in the immediate postoperative period. The dose used will need to be tailored to the age, weight and physical state of the patient. It is probably better to use smaller and more frequent doses. Adverse effects of opiates in the elderly are respiration depression, drowsiness, nausea, confusion and constipation.
- *Non-steroidal anti-inflammatory*: These drugs may be given orally, rectally or intramuscularly. Whilst their use is attractive because they have no effects on respiration, concern has been expressed that they may have an adverse effect on renal function and increase the risk of excessive bleeding at surgery, especially in combination with low-molecular-weight heparin.

Preoperative traction

Traditional teaching has been to apply traction to the injured limb prior to surgery in the belief that this reduces the amount of pain. Three recent randomized trials have however shown traction to be of no benefit to the patient in reducing the amount of pain or affecting the ease of fracture reduction at the time of surgery.

There appears to be therefore no reason for the routine use of traction. However, opinions are divided as to whether traction should be used for a displaced intracapsular fracture which is to be treated by reduction and internal fixation. It may be that traction will reduce movement at the fracture site and prevent further damage to capsular vessels.

Correction of hypovolaemia

Dehydration and hypovolaemia may occur prior to surgery. This can be caused by a number of factors – the lack of oral fluid intake following the injury and during transfer to and assessment in hospital. The use of opiate analgesia may potentiate dehydrating by causing nausea and vomiting. A variable amount of blood volume will be lost from the fracture site. Blood loss is greater for extracapsular fractures where the loss from a comminuted trochanteric fracture frequently exceeds one litre. Intracapsular fractures result in only a small blood loss, as the fracture surfaces are small and contained within the joint capsule which has a tamponade effect.

If anaesthesia and surgery are undertaken before correction of hypovolaemia, hypotension will occur with an increase in mortality. It is therefore essential to administer intravenous fluids prior to surgery. Careful fluid balance is however essential for hip fracture patients as there is frequently a fine balance between correct hydration and over-hydration leading to cardiac failure.

Hypothermia

Hypothermia may occur following a fracture, especially if the patient is unable to summon assistance. Hypothermia may also be present prior to the fall and has been implicated in the aetiology of hip fractures. Other related factors which may be relevant are low body mass and excessive alcohol consumption. Diagnosis of hypothermia requires a low-reading rectal thermometer and treatment is by gradual rewarming. Cardiac arrhythmias may occur and surgery should be delayed until body temperature is normal.

Timing of surgery

This is a controversial subject. Some surgeons have argued that a hip fracture is a surgical emergency. These patients should be operated on immediately, before complications develop. Conversely, others have stated that there should be a few days of preoperative assessment and resuscitation before surgery. Evidence from the literature is conflicting, though the following recommendations can be made:

Table 3.4 Justifiable reasons for delaying hip fracture surgery

Anaemia (haemoglobin less than 100 g/l)

Uraemia (urea above 10 mmol/l)

Severe electrolyte imbalance

Hypovolaemia

Congestive cardiac failure

Severe hypertension

Rapid atrial fibrillation, or other correctable cardiac arrhythmia

Chest infection

Acute exacerbation of chronic chest condition

Unstable diabetes mellitus

1 Surgery need not be performed as an immediate 'out-of-hours' procedure, thereby allowing some hours for preoperative assessment and resuscitation.
2 For the majority of patients, delaying surgery beyond 24 hours from admission will result in a small but progressive increase in complications associated with bed rest, such as bronchopneumonia, pressure sores and thrombosis.
3 In approximately 10% of patients, preoperative assessment will reveal a medical condition which is better corrected or improved prior to surgery. Such conditions are listed in Table 3.4.
4 Chronic pathology that cannot be improved should not be used as a reason for delaying surgery.
5 For intracapsular fractures that are to be treated by internal fixation, there is some evidence that early surgical intervention reduces the risk of non-union and avascular necrosis. This is discussed further in Chapter 5.

Prophylaxis against thromboembolism

Hip fracture patients are at high risk of developing thrombotic complications, regardless of the type of treatment. Classical physical signs are present in only 2–4% of patients. If routine venography is performed then the incidence of venous thrombosis has been reported to be between 30 and 90% and an autopsy study has reported an incidence of 83%.

Prophylactic measures to reduce the high risk of thrombotic complications are therefore essential. Pharmacological measures that may be used are listed in Table 3.5.

To be most effective pharmacological measures should be started as soon as possible after admission and preferably before surgery. Of these drugs, the four most commonly used are heparin, warfarin, aspirin and dextran.

Heparin

This is the most commonly used method and has been the subject of the greatest number of clinical studies. Heparin can reduce the incidence of thrombosis, as demonstrated by venography, from 46% to 28%. Standard or unfractionated heparin is given in a dose of 5000 units subcutaneously, twice or three times daily, starting as soon as possible after admission and continuing for 5–14 days after surgery.

Recently, low-molecular-weight heparins have been introduced. These offer the convenience of a once-daily dosage and may be slightly more effective than unfractionated heparin.

Table 3.5 Pharmacological measures used in hip fracture patients to reduce the incidence of thromboembolism

Heparin
Dextran
Warfarin
Phenindione
Ancrod
Aspirin
Dipyridamole
Non-steroidal anti-inflammatory
Hydroxychloroquine
Dihydroergotamine
Streptokinase

Warfarin

Oral anticoagulation using warfarin is the most effective pharmacological method of reducing thromboembolic complications. This is achieved at the price of an increased risk of haemorrhagic complications, which tend to be more common in the elderly and may even be fatal. Strict attention to monitoring is therefore required to maintain the international normalized ratio (INR) at between 2 and 3 times normal. If there is no delay to surgery, treatment may be started in the perioperative period. Alternatively, therapy is begun on admission and the INR checked immediately before surgery. Other problems with warfarin are its potential interactions with other drugs. These factors make the use of warfarin following a hip fracture unattractive, despite its proven efficacy.

Aspirin

Oral aspirin in low dosage (75–300 mg daily) affects platelet function. Its efficacy after hip fracture has been the subject of only a limited number of studies with conflicting results. Aspirin does have the advantages of simplicity of administration and a low incidence of adverse effects.

Dextran

Clinical studies of dextran 70 indicate that it has similar efficacy to warfarin. The optimum dosage is uncertain but most studies recommend 500 ml on diagnosis, 500 ml during surgery and then on alternative days for 3 days. Potential complications of dextran are fluid overload, interference with blood crossmatching and anaphylactic reactions.

Mechanical measures

Mechanical devices are available to compress the calf or foot. They need to be used before, during and for the days following surgery. Theoretically these methods are attractive because of the absence of adverse effects, but their effectiveness after hip fracture is at present unproven. Antiembolism stockings have been used but are frequently found by hip fracture patients to be difficult to put on and may be uncomfortable to wear.

Summary of recommended thromboembolic prophylaxis

Current opinion suggests that in those patients in whom there are no contraindications, pharmacological measures should be used. Heparin is most commonly used; alternatives are dextran, aspirin or warfarin. Mechanical measures, if available, may also be used.

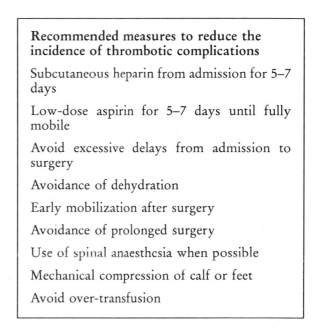

Recommended measures to reduce the incidence of thrombotic complications

Subcutaneous heparin from admission for 5–7 days

Low-dose aspirin for 5–7 days until fully mobile

Avoid excessive delays from admission to surgery

Avoidance of dehydration

Early mobilization after surgery

Avoidance of prolonged surgery

Use of spinal anaesthesia when possible

Mechanical compression of calf or feet

Avoid over-transfusion

Antibiotic prophylaxis and prevention of wound sepsis

Wound sepsis following hip fracture surgery is a potentially devastating complication. A high priority should be paid to preventive measures. It should be possible to reduce the incidence of deep wound sepsis to almost zero, with meticulous attention to the following details.

Preoperatively

Elderly hip fracture patients frequently have potential sources of sepsis such as leg sores, pressure areas and bacteriuria. These factors should not be considered as a contraindication to surgery, but wherever possible active infection should be treated prior to surgery.

Strict theatre discipline

Ideally hip fracture surgery should be carried out in a designated orthopaedic theatre, with appropriately trained theatre personnel. Unnecessary movement of theatre staff should be restricted and strict attention must be paid to asepsis at all times.

Operative technique

Appropriate skin preparation, towelling and minimal handling of tissues during surgery should be encouraged. Measures such as the use of plastic occlusive drapes and a double-glove technique are recommended. The implant itself should not be handled and should not come into contact with the patient's skin. Excessive tissue dissection and prolonged surgery should also be avoided. At the end of the operation the skin should be closed with careful and atraumatic apposition of the skin edges, to promote early skin healing. The use of absorbable subcuticular sutures is advocated.

Use of drains

The value of closed suction drainage following hip fracture surgery is debatable. The theoretical advantage of a drain is to reduce the extent of haematoma formation within the wound, which may act as a potential culture medium for organisms. Disadvantages are that organisms will migrate from the skin along the drain and this may increase sepsis.

The limited number of clinical studies on this aspect of hip fracture surgery have produced conflicting results. The trend is for there to be no demonstrable benefit from the routine use of drains. For intracapsular fracture, whether treated by internal fixation or hemiarthroplasty, blood loss is generally minimal and a drain is probably of little benefit. For fixation of an extracapsular fracture there tends to be a greater blood loss from the fracture site which is not preventable. The use of a closed suction drain may therefore be justifiable for a comminuted extracapsular fracture.

Prophylactic antibiotics

Clinical studies indicate that the use of prophylactic antibiotics reduces the incidence of deep wound infection from approximately 3% to 1%. Drugs which have been used include cefuroxime, cephalothin, cefazolin, flucloxacillin and nafacillin. The first dose should be given intravenously at the beginning of surgery and a further one to three

---

Summary of preoperative requirements for hip fracture patients

Diagnose and classify the fracture

Assess the patient for other injuries

Note the presence of other associated illnesses

If other treatable disorders are present (Table 3.4), correct as appropriate

Provide adequate analgesia

Correct hypovolaemia with intravenous fluids

Perform routine preoperative investigations

Prescribe thromboembolic prophylaxis

Minimize time spent in casualty and in transfers to reduce the risk of pressure sores

Inform patient and relatives of the diagnosis and proposed treatment, along with plans for discharge

Minimize delays from admission to operation, but avoid 'out-of-hours' surgery

Perform operation in a designated orthopaedic theatre with appropriate support staff

Use prophylactic antibiotics

Use spinal anaesthesia if possible

Ensure surgery is performed by an experienced surgeon to minimize complications

doses given over the next 24 hours. Commencing the antibiotics too early before surgery risks colonization with resistant organisms. The use of more prolonged courses of antibiotics has an increased risk of adverse effects for no additional benefit.

Anaesthesia for hip fracture surgery

A variety of methods are available for hip fracture surgery, but in the majority of cases the choice is between general or regional (spinal) anaesthesia. This question has been the subject of a number of studies, many of them randomized. The overall conclusion from the literature is that spinal anaesthesia results in a small reduction in the immediate postoperative mortality, but after 1 month there is no difference in mortality for spinal or general anaesthesia.

Spinal anaesthesia is associated with a small reduction in the incidence of thromboembolic complications and bleeding at the time of surgery. This is due to peripheral vasodilation and increased blood flow to the limbs. It is reasonable to conclude that spinal anaesthesia is marginally preferable to generally anaesthesia.

Key references on medical assessment

Collin C, Wade DT, Davies S, Horne V. The Barthel ADL index: a reliability study. *Int Disabil Studies* 1988; 10:61–63.

Parker MJ, Palmer CR. A new mobility score for predicting mortality after hip fracture. *J Bone Joint Surg* 1993; **75–B**:797–798.

Qureshi KN, Hodkinson HM. Evaluation of a ten-question mental test in the institutionalized elderly. *Age Ageing* 1974; **3**:152–157.

Thorngren K-G, Ceder L, Svensson K. Predicting results of rehabilitation after hip fracture; a ten-year follow-up study. *Clin Orthop* 1993; **287**:76–81.

White BL, Fisher WD, Laurin CA. Rate of mortality for elderly patients after fracture of the hip in the 1980s. *J Bone Joint Surg* 1987; **69–A**:1335–1340.

Key references on preparation for theatre

Anderson GH, Harper WM, Connelly CD, Badham J, Goodrich N, Gregg PJ. Pre-operative skin traction for fractures of the proximal femur: a randomized prospective trial. *J Bone Joint Surg* 1993; **75–B**:794–796.

Finsen F, Børset M, Buvik GE, Hauke I. Preoperative traction in patients with hip fractures. *Injury* 1992; **23**:242–244.

Gillespie WJ, Awal KH, Farrar MJ, Handoll HHG, McBirnie J, Milne AA, Tytherleigh-Strong G. Prophylaxis against deep vein thrombosis and pulmonary embolism in hip fracture surgery. In: Gillespie WJ, Madhok R, Swiontkowski M, Robinson CM, Murray GD (eds) Musculoskeletal injuries Module of The Cochrane Library [database on disk and CDROM]. The Cochrane Collaboration; Oxford: Update software: 1996. BMJ publishing group, London.

Needoff M, Radford P, Langstaff R. Preoperative traction for hip fractures in the elderly: a clinical trial. *Injury* 1993; **24**:317–318.

Parker MJ, Pryor GA, Myles JW. The value of a special surgical team in preventing complications in the treatment of hip fractures. *Int Orthop* 1994; **18**:184–188.

Sevitt S, Gallagher N. Venous thrombosis and pulmonary embolism clinico-pathological study in injured and burned patients. *Br J Surg* 1961; **48**:475–489.

4

Use of the fracture table and image intensifier

The correct use of the fracture table (traction table) is an integral part of internal fixation of hip fractures. The patient needs to be correctly prepared and positioned to reduce the fracture and at the same time allow for the image intensifier to take X-rays in two planes. A biplane image intensifier, if available, will facilitate this. Particular points to note are the following:

1 Ensure all the necessary equipment is available prior to commencing the operation.
2 Supervise transferring the patient to the fracture table, as the patient is at risk of falling from the narrow operating table. To reduce the risk of pressure sores, padding should be applied to any areas of pressure such as around the feet, sacrum and groin. For an intracapsular fracture the injured leg must be treated with great care to prevent fracture displacement occurring or damage to the retinacular vessels. If traction is being used for a displaced intracapsular fracture it should be maintained during transfer of the patient.
3 Position the pelvis so that the injured hip is lying clear of the table.
4 Abduct the uninjured leg as much as possible and fix this in a gutter support, stirrup or with the foot fixed in a boot, attached to the table limb support (Fig. 4.1). Positioning of the image intensifier is often easier if the hip and knee are flexed

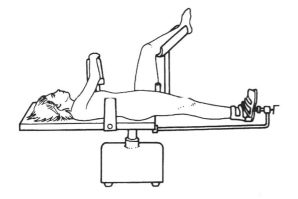
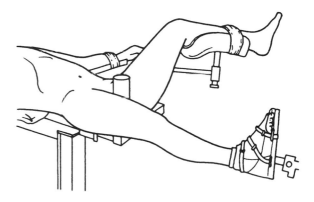

Fig. 4.1 Recommended positioning of the patient on the fracture table.

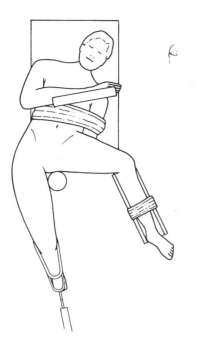

Fig. 4.2   For an intramedullary nailing the trunk needs to be flexed away from the fracture site and the injured leg slightly adducted to allow the nail to be inserted. The table should be tilted slightly to raise the fracture side to improve access. A Steinmann pin in the distal femur allowing the knee to flex may assist reduction.

to 90°. Avoid excessive force on the uninjured leg which could cause an additional fracture.

5   To counteract any traction applied to the limb a perineal post is used or alternatively a sling around the groin. The groin post may unfortunately reduce the quality of the X-ray images on the lateral view. Frequently, for intracapsular fractures, the post can be omitted as the amount of longitudinal traction is minimal.

6   Place the injured leg in the supporting boot, attached to the table limb support. Ensure that the support will not obscure the anteroposterior (AP) view of the fractured hip. The exact method of fracture reduction depends on the type of fracture and this is discussed in Chapters 5–7.

7   The surgeon must be familiar with the mechanism by which the boot is attached to the table. The fracture table allows longitudinal traction to be applied to the limb, whilst at the same time allowing the

foot to be locked in the appropriate position of rotation.

8   The degree of rotation of the injured limb will depend on the site and degree of displacement of the fracture. For undisplaced intracapsular fractures and trochanteric fracture 10° of internal rotation is best as this brings the femoral neck horizontal to the ground. For displaced intracapsular fractures full internal rotation is generally required (see chapter 5). A rough guide is the patella, the anterior surface of which should be facing the ceiling.

9   A side support or stout strapping should be used to hold the arm adducted and out of the way and stabilize the trunk, preventing the patient being pulled off the table.

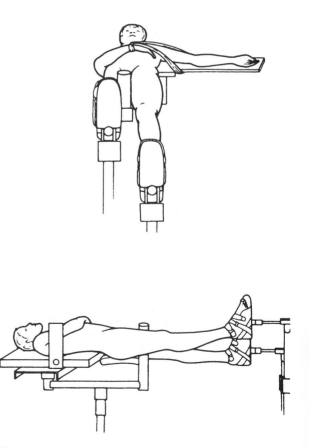

Fig. 4.3   Alternative positioning in the presence of severe limitation of movement of the uninjured hip.

10 If an intramedullary procedure is being undertaken then the trunk should be flexed away from the fracture side to give cleared access to the area above the greater trochanter. The uninjured leg needs to be abducted out of the way as much as possible whilst the injured leg cannot be abducted but needs to be placed in a position of slight adduction to allow access for the nail to be inserted into the greater trochanter (Fig. 4.2). Tilting the table to the side away from the fracture may also improve access to the trochanteric region.

11 Occasionally it is necessary to insert a Steinmann pin into the distal femur to allow the knee of the injured leg to be flexed. This can be useful in subtrochanteric fractures if there is flexion of the distal fragment preventing fracture reduction (Fig. 4.2).

12 Severe limitation of movement of the contralateral hip will occasionally prevent the

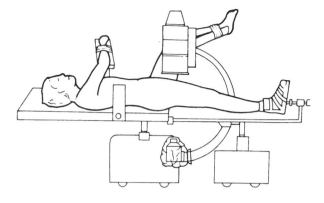

Fig. 4.5 Correct positioning for the image intensifier for the anteroposterior view.

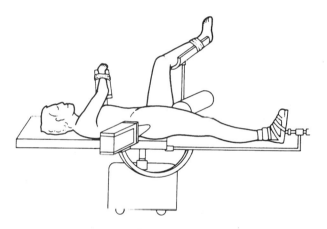

Fig. 4.6 Correct positioning for the image intensifier for the lateral view. The camera unit should be placed as close to the groin as possible but also angled as close to 90° as possible to the injured leg. This is particularly important if an intramedullary nailing procedure is being undertaken to allow the surgeon access to the trochanteric region.

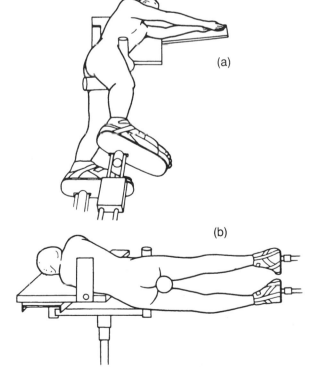

Fig. 4.4 (a, b) Alternative positioning for intramedullary nailing.

uninjured leg being abducted. In this situation the position shown in Figure 4.3 can be used. Both hips are in slight abduction, with the injured hip slightly flexed and the contralateral hip slightly extended. This positioning can be used for intramedullary nailing of subtrochanteric fractures where visualization of the femoral head is not paramount.

13 Occasionally a lateral position may be used for an intramedullary nailing procedure (Fig. 4.4). This gives better access to insert the nail at the greater trochanteric, but it is harder to obtain a good X-ray

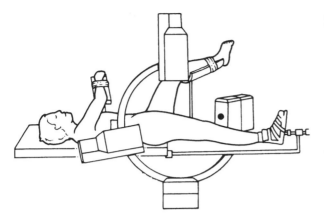

Fig. 4.7 A biplanar image intensifier enables the anteroposterior and lateral radiographs to be taken simultaneously.

picture of the femoral head as both hip joints tend to be superimposed on each other.

14 Check the AP radiograph to confirm adequate fracture reduction. To obtain the best picture ensure there are no intervening objects between the patient and the image intensifier. The image intensifier unit should be lowered as much as possible, so that there is minimal distance between the anterior thigh and the camera unit (Fig. 4.5).

15 Check the lateral radiograph. To obtain the clearest picture, the C arm of the image intensifier should be positioned so the camera unit is as close to the patient's groin as possible. In addition the unit needs to be angled as shown in Figure 4.6. This reduces the amount of intervening soft tissue.

16 A biplane image intensifier may be used if available (Fig. 4.7). This has the advantage of allowing AP and lateral X-ray views to be taken simultaneously, thereby saving time. It is also easier to screen a pin or guidewire into position using the two views and because there is no need to move the machine once positioned, there is less risk of jeopardizing the sterile draping.

When using a biplanar image intensifier, advance the G stand by pushing it from the foot up around the fractured leg to the hip area. For a dynamic hip screw or parallel screw fixation, position it with an angle of about 135° to the longitudinal axis of the leg, with the lateral view source in the groin and this X-ray tube at approximately 45° to the trunk of the patient. This results in the camera unit for the lateral view being against the patient's

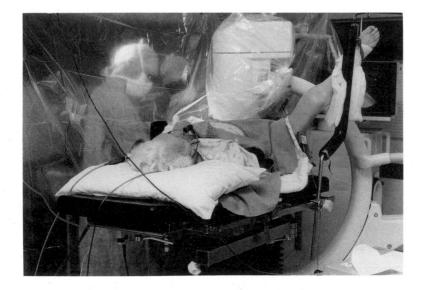

Fig. 4.8   The use of a sterile plastic isolation drape is recommended with the fracture table.

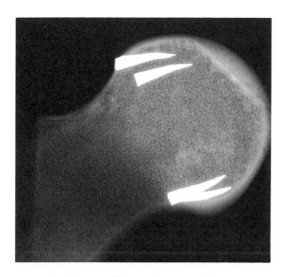

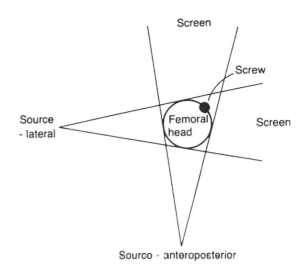

Fig. 4.10 Method by which the tip of an implant may incorrectly appear to be within the femoral head.

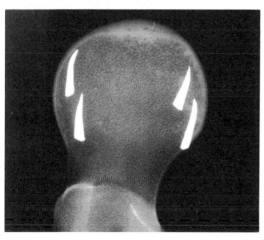

trunk during the operation, with the surgeon standing to the caudal side of the camera. For an intramedullary nail fixation, the G arm is placed as near to 90° to the patient's leg. The camera unit for the lateral X-ray is caudal to the surgeon, who stands between the camera unit and the patient's trunk.

17 If an intramedullary nailing procedure is being undertaken then the image intensifier needs to be set up to allow access to the superior trochanteric area. For the lateral view the C arm should be used in as near a transverse position as possible (Fig. 4.6). Check before draping that the surgeon can access the area proximal to the greater trochanter whilst still obtaining AP and lateral X-rays. Depending on the type of nail to be used it will probably be necessary to visualize the entire femur on both the AP and lateral radiographs, so ensure the leg supports do not obscure the AP view.

18 The skin is then prepared with an aseptic solution and dried. A large plastic isolation drape may then be used to isolate the sterile operative area from other theatre staff (Fig. 4.8). A transparent drape is preferable as it allows the surgeon to check that the C arm is correctly positioned.

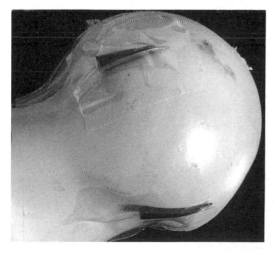

Fig. 4.9 The tips of these metal markers appear on the radiographs to be within the bone, but in practice they are outside.

19 When positioning the tip of the implant close to the subchondral bone, remember that an implant may appear to be within the femoral head on the both the AP and lateral views, but actually to have penetrated the femoral head (Fig. 4.9). Why this may occur is illustrated in Figure 4.10, demonstrating that peripheral placement on both the AP and lateral views considerably increases the risk of undetected joint penetration. Placing the implant within the centre of the femoral head is therefore preferred, as it eliminates the risk of inadvertent joint penetration occurring.

Key references

Bagga TK. Comparative evaluation of the two positions used for imaging of trochanteric fractures. *Injury* 1994; 25:653–654.

Stewart WG. The image intensifier in hip fracture surgery. *Orthop Clin North Am* 1974; 5:933–938.

5

Internal fixation of intracapsular fractures

The internal fixation of intracapsular fractures involves inserting parallel pins or screws (usually two or three) within the femoral neck and head, parallel to the longitudinal axis of the femoral neck. The positioning of the osteosynthesis material is intended to allow impaction of the femoral neck fracture when the patient is weight-bearing. It is the aim of the orthopaedic surgeon to stabilize the fracture so that direct weight-bearing and walking can start as early as the day after the operation.

Indications

As discussed in Chapter 2, this method of treatment is recommended for the majority of undisplaced and minimally displaced intracapsular fractures, and should also be considered for displaced intracapsular fractures. However, within these groups of patients there will be specific fracture types for which arthroplasty may be a more appropriate form of treatment. These are listed here and discussed further in Chapter 2.

Timing of surgery

Undisplaced intracapsular fractures

For undisplaced fractures early surgery will allow aspiration of any haematoma within the joint. This may reduce the risk of avascular necrosis caused by ischaemia from a tamponade effect on the intracapsular vessels. The evidence for any benefit is not sufficient to merit out-of-hours surgery, but preferably surgery should be undertaken within 24 h of admission.

Intracapsular fractures in which arthroplasty may be more suitable than internal fixation

Displaced intracapsular fractures in the elderly

Displaced intracapsular fractures with a delay in diagnosis

Displaced intracapsular fractures in patients with rheumatoid arthritis

Intracapsular fractures secondary to Paget's disease

Intracapsular fractures secondary to malignancy

Intracapsular fractures associated with metabolic bone disease

Hip fracture with coexistent arthritis of the hip

Displaced intracapsular fractures

The argument in favour of early surgery (within 6–8 hours), for displaced intracapsular fractures is that it will allow straightening of capsular vessels around the fracture site. This may reduce the subsequent risk of non-union and avascular necrosis. Studies to date have given conflicting results and therefore the general advice is the same as for undisplaced fractures. The exception is with a young patient (less than 50 years), where preservation of the femoral head is paramount and immediate surgery may be justifiable.

Once more than 48 hours have elapsed from injury there is a progressive increase in the risk of healing complications following internal fixation. By one week it will generally not be possible to achieve a closed reduction of the fracture and internal fixation alone should not be undertaken. In these circumstances the surgeon must consider whether an arthroplasty would be preferable or to perform an open fracture reduction, possibly combined with a revascularization procedure to the femoral head.

Choice of implant

Originally femoral neck fractures were nailed with a flanged nail. This method was introduced by Smith-Petersen in 1931. He applied open reduction of the fracture. Sven Johansson in 1932 pioneered closed nailing by cannulating the Smith-Peterson nail, which allowed insertion of a guidewire, and nailing over this after a check X-ray. Since then over 100 different modifications of nails, screws and pins have been used.

During the last decade the importance of low-traumatic technique has been emphasized to preserve the remaining circulation to the femoral head. Pre-drilling is used and hammering avoided. It has also been shown that hammering on the greater trochanter to compress the fracture will impair the circulation to the femoral head. The best way to compress the fracture is through the patient's own muscle forces and by weight-bearing. This has led

to the use of parallel pins or screws to allow axial compression along the axis of the femoral neck perpendicular to the fracture line.

To reduce the risk of fixation failure, osteosynthesis material with either threaded screws or a hook that can be pressed out through a central canal has been developed. To facilitate parallel positioning most devices are cannulated and have instruments to enable parallel placement.

Opinions differ between orthopaedic surgeons as to the choice of implant and there is conflicting evidence within the literature. The most commonly used methods of fixation are two or three parallel cancellous screws (Fig. 5.4), two parallel pins (Fig. 5.12) or a dynamic hip screw (Fig. 5.14).

Reduction of the fracture

Clearly no reduction is appropriate for undisplaced intracapsular fractures. Furthermore no attempt should be made to disimpact an impacted intracapsular fracture. All displaced fractures must be reduced prior to fixation.

As discussed in Chapter 2, an intracapsular fracture may appear undisplaced on the anteroposterior (AP) radiograph, whilst there has been some opening of the fracture line on the lateral radiograph (See Fig. 2.9). In such cases reduction of the fracture is readily achieved by internal rotation of the leg. This manoeuvre is best achieved whilst screening the fracture on the lateral X-ray.

Closed reduction

The position of the patient on the fracture table is described in Chapter 4. The surgeon should supervise the transfer of the patient to the fracture table to guard against undue and excessive movement of the fractured hip. The blood circulation to the femoral head via the capsular vessels along the femoral neck is vulnerable. Sudden forceful movements of the hip during reduction or excessive traction

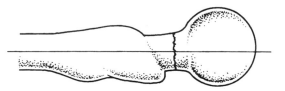

Fig. 5.1 Internal rotation of the foot should result in the femoral head, neck and shaft all appearing in a straight line with no residual angulation at the fracture site.

causing fracture diastasis may jeopardize femoral head circulation. The fracture is usually reduced by applying minimal traction to the outstretched leg, followed by internal rotation. These manoeuvres should be checked throughout the procedure in both the lateral and AP radiographs using an image intensifier, with good resolution facilities.

The reduction manoeuvre is begun by using the fracture table to apply gentle traction to the leg progressively whilst checking in the AP radiograph. Traction is applied until the medial parts of the femoral neck, the calcar region, are approximated with anatomical contact between the bone ends. Next the lateral view is obtained and the foot is rotated inwards until the dorsal angulation in the femoral neck fracture has been counteracted. This part of the manoeuvre can be likened to closing an open book. The aim is to restore the alignment of the femoral neck such that a straight line can be drawn to bisect the femoral head, trochanteric region and shaft (Fig. 5.1).

It is essential that there is no residual angulation at the fracture site as this will increase the risk of re-displacement of the fracture. The foot frequently needs to be placed in excess of 90° internal rotation to achieve reduction. Over-reduction of a displaced intracapsular fracture by internal rotation is rare as reduction is being hinged by the soft tissues, particularly the ligament of Weitbrecht. The reduction manoeuvre can be compared to that of a Colles fracture, where the fracture is reduced on the intact volar soft-tissue hinge and over-reduction is very unusual (Fig. 5.2).

Small corrections with ab- adduction and sometimes elevation of the leg may also be needed to obtain anatomical reduction. With excessive internal rotation the plane of the femoral neck shifts from a superolateral to inferomedial direction. This may distort the appearance of the femoral neck and make interpretation of X-ray more difficult.

Throughout this internal rotation manoeuvre a couple of check X-rays in the AP projection should be performed, to check that no gross malposition is appearing. Following this reduction manoeuvre it is advisable to slacken the traction somewhat. This allows some impaction to occur at the fracture site and reduces the risk of the femoral head rotation during surgery.

Other reduction manoeuvres, such as those described by Leadbetter (1933) and Flynn (1974), involve a more forceful twisting manoeuvre. These may disrupt the remaining

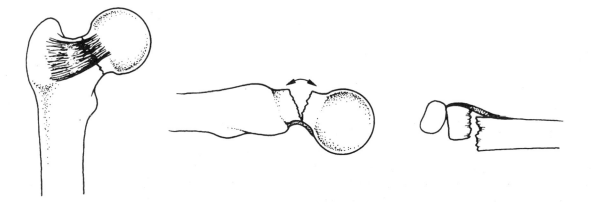

Fig. 5.2 Reduction of an intracapsular fracture is akin to that of a Colles fracture using a soft-tissue hinge.

circulation to the femoral head. They are probably best avoided and only used for those fractures where reduction is not possible by the methods described above.

For the Leadbetter manoeuvre, the surgeon stands on the side of the fractured hip, holding the affected leg. An assistant stabilizes the pelvis by pressing down on both anterior iliac spines. The limb is first flexed 90° at the hip and the knee. Traction is then applied to the femur in a vertical direction. While maintaining traction the leg is then fully internally rotated and brought into extension and some abduction. The foot is then secured to the fracture table.

The quality of fracture reduction can be assessed by the Garden alignment index (Fig. 5.3). An anatomical reduction is 160°/180° (Fig. 5.4). An acceptable angle for the AP view is between 160° and 180°, in fact, a slight valgus position may be preferable. A varus position is not acceptable. For the lateral angulation, the nearer the angle is to 180° the better.

With the described careful stepwise traction and inward rotation, supplemented with necessary ab- or adduction, most femoral neck fractures can be reduced. The goal is to achieve an anatomical reduction, but occasionally a less than ideal position has to be accepted and the implant inserted. For such cases the fixation should be tested post-operatively by allowing the patient to weight-bear. After some days a check X-ray can be performed. If an early re-displacement of the fracture appears, a planned secondary arthroplasty can be performed within some days or weeks.

Open reduction

The pioneers of femoral neck fracture surgery in the early 1930s used a large exposure of the fracture, open reduction and nailing under direct vision. Bone grafting with a free fibula graft and later with vascularized grafts, such as rotation of the bony insertion of the quadratus femoris muscle, has since been described.

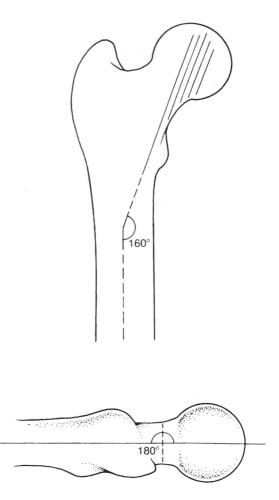

Fig. 5.3 The Garden alignment index used to assess fracture reduction. An anatomical reduction is 160°/180°.

With the introduction of the fracture table and X-ray image intensification, open reduction is now only rarely indicated. Arthrotomy may cause additional damage to capsular vessels and arguments that arthrotomy is required to confirm fracture reduction or aspirate the hip are no longer tenable.

Open reduction should therefore only be used when preservation of the femoral head is paramount and one of the following situations is present:

1 Inability to obtain an adequate closed reduction.
2 Fractures more than 1 week old.

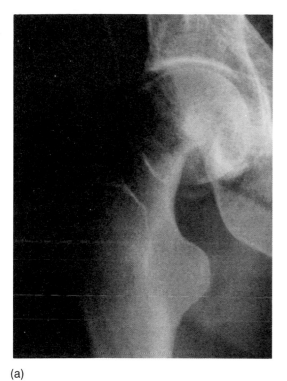

(a)

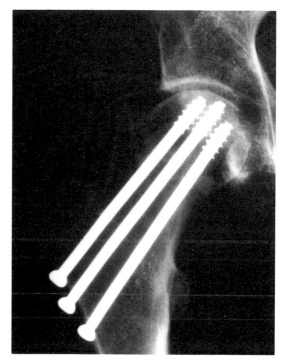

(c)

(b)

(d)

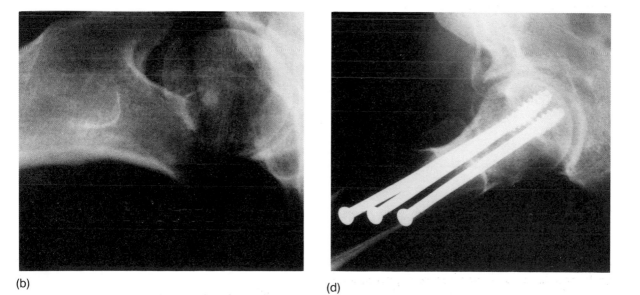

Fig. 5.4(a–d)   Anteroposterior and lateral X-rays of correct reduction of a displaced intracapsular fracture.

3 Early re-displacement following internal fixation.

For the second and third of these indications it may be preferable to combine the procedure with insertion of a vascularized muscle/bone pedicle graft into the fracture site. Descriptions of vascularized pedicle grafts are beyond the scope of this book. The reader is referred to the description by Meyers of a posterior approach for a graft based on quadratus femoris, the anterior approach based on the gluteus medius by De Das, or that for a graft based on the sartorius muscle by Baksi.

If open reduction only is required, a limited anterior approach is conventionally used, as described originally by Smith-Petersen. A posterior approach has the advantage of giving better access to the fracture site, but increased risk of damaging capsular vessels. A full operative description of open reduction of an intracapsular fracture is beyond the scope of this book; it is a demanding operation and should not be undertaken by an inexperienced surgeon.

Aspiration of the hip

Bleeding from the fracture site into the joint capsule may result in pressures high enough to impair the circulation in the small arteries situated subperiostally along the femoral neck – a bleeding tamponade effect. A tense haematoma within the joint is more common in undisplaced fractures, where the joint capsule usually has not ruptured. This may be suspected clinically when there is excessive pain in the groin area, particularly on rotating the hip. For displaced fractures, the joint capsule is frequently ruptured, allowing blood to escape into the soft tissue around the hip joint.

Theoretically, therefore, any haematoma should be aspirated as soon as possible, even in the Accident and Emergency department. Clinical studies to date are nevertheless

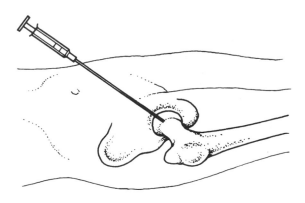

Fig. 5.5   Aspiration of the hip using a needle inserted in a posterior and medial direction under X-ray control.

unclear as to how beneficial hip joint aspiration is to the eventual outcome, particularly to the risk of subsequent avascular necrosis.

The haematoma is conventionally evacuated by a needle inserted under X-ray image intensification. The needle is preferably inserted semivertically from the anterolateral area and directed inferior-medially (Fig. 5.5). The femoral artery is palpated to lie clearly medial to the injection site. The route of the needle is verified with the image intensifier. Usually a palpable resistance is felt when the needle penetrates the capsule. Any haematoma which is normally 2–10 ml in volume can then be aspirated.

Positioning of the osteosynthesis device

Two hook pins or screws

Examples of these are Hansson hook pins, von Bahr, Uppsala, Ullevaal and Garden screws. They are usually about 7 mm in diameter and inserted parallel to each other. The aim is to create a three-point fixation, where the first point is the entry hole through the firm lateral cortical bone, the second point is the pin lying on the calcar inferiorly or posteriorly, and the third at the subchondral bone plate.

The lateral skin incision extends distally from a point about 2 cm distal to the greater

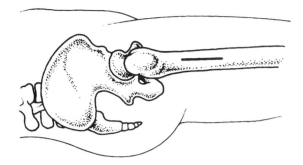

Fig. 5.6   Lateral skin incision.

trochanter for a length of about 5 cm (Fig. 5.6). The exact position of the incision may be best located using a guidewire or similar radiopaque object on the skin surface and screening in the AP view. A wire can be held against the patient's side while screening in the lateral view should be in the centre of the femoral head, neck and shaft.

With experience the femoral surface need not be exposed, the guidewires and pins being passed percutaneously through the intervening soft tissues to the bone. A Kirschner wire is normally used as a guide in the femur and then the cannulated pin or screw is positioned over the wire. It is best to try and position the lower screw first. The entry point is determined by holding a guidewire over the patient's skin and screening on the AP image. The guidewire should run from the femoral head along the calcar to cross the lateral cortex at the level of the middle-lower part of the lesser trochanter (Fig. 5.7). If the screw is inserted distal to this point there is an increased risk of fracture of the femur around the distal screw.

The initial hole created by drilling the Kirschner guidewire through the lateral cortex has a strong guiding capacity and if incorrect it is difficult to reposition the Kirschner wire. One way to overcome this is to drill a slightly larger hole in the lateral cortex and then the Kirschner wire can be positioned through this more precisely.

Some surgeons prefer to use the definite drill hole first without a guidewire but this requires some experience. To avoid the drill slipping, first drill through one cortex into the medullary canal at a right angle to the longitudinal axis of the femur. Then with the bit continuing to rotate, angle the drill towards the femoral head. The drill tip is slowly advanced up along the calcar femorale into the femoral head, to the joint line. The position is repeatedly checked on X-rays in the AP and lateral plane. To ensure the correct direction of the drilling, a Kirschner wire can be placed outside the patient on the draping over the femoral head. Alternatively one may be placed immediately anterior to the femoral neck (Fig. 5.8).

On the lateral view the guidewire should appear within the centre of the femoral head and neck (Fig. 5.9). It is important to realize that the forces during weight-bearing tend to compress the fracture further in an anatomical position. If the fixation device is not placed parallel with the long axis of the femoral neck, weight-bearing may lead to re-displacement of the fracture.

The second guidewire is then placed in a proximal position parallel to the first one. A guide instrument is frequently available to facilitate this placement. This is usually a

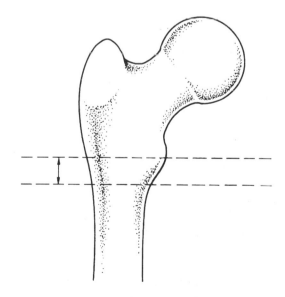

Fig. 5.7   The site of insertion of the distal screw or pin is level with the mid to lower part of the lesser trochanter.

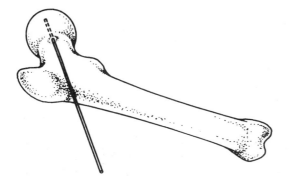

Fig. 5.8   A guidewire placed anterior to the femoral neck may be used to aid guidewire placement.

block with predrilled parallel holes and utilizes the first guidewire. On the lateral X-ray the second pin should be positioned to rest on the dorsal (posterior) cortex of the femoral neck, thereby resisting dorsal angulation at the fracture during weight-bearing (Fig. 5.10).

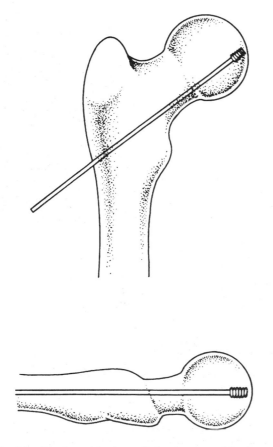

Fig. 5.9   Ideal positioning of the lower guidewire or drill on the anteroposterior and lateral radiographs.

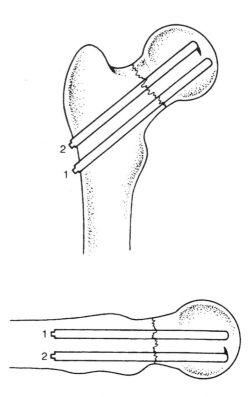

Fig. 5.10   Correct positioning of two parallel Hansson pins.

For this posterior positioning it is prudent not to place the pin or screw too close to the joint surface. Otherwise there will be a risk of inadvertent joint penetration which may not be apparent on the X-ray.

Once each guidewire is positioned the required length of the pin or screw is determined. There are frequently measurements marked on the special drills so the part protruding from the guide can be directly read off. In some screw systems an additional allowance has to be made for the length of the screw head which will be protruding from the femur. Screws which protrude excessively from the lateral femoral cortex should be avoided. Subsequent impaction of the fracture will result in excessive lateral protrusion which may cause a painful swelling. The screws or pins are then placed either over the guidewires or through the predrilled holes. The final position of the screws should be checked on both AP and lateral radiographs (Figs 5.11 and 5.12).

<table>
<tr><td>

Correct positioning of two screws

Distal screw entry point in lateral cortex level with the middle to lower part of the lesser trochanter

Distal screw lying just superior to the calcar on the anteroposterior (AP) radiograph

Distal screw lying centrally in the lateral X-ray

Proximal screw centrally placed on the AP X-ray

Proximal screw touching posterior cortex on the lateral X-ray

Tip of both screws about 5 mm from the joint line

</td></tr>
</table>

One or two sutures in the fascia lata are usually required to aid wound closure. This may diminish the feeling of pressure against the skin when the patient is lying on the operated side. The skin edges should be accurately closed with absorbable subcuticular sutures.

Three or more screws

A number of manufacturers make thinner screws of 6–7 mm in diameter such as those of the Gouffon, AO or Asnis type. Many of these self-tapping screws are cannulated to enable them to be passed over a guidewire. Each type of screw has different lengths and types of screw threads, but it is difficult to be sure what is the optimum configuration.

When three screws are used, the inferior one is usually inserted resting on the calcar. For the other two proximal screws, one is slightly anterior and the other is placed to touch the posterior cortex. The lowest screw should not be inserted distal to the lower border of the lesser trochanter. This will avoid the risk of causing a subtrochanteric stress fracture.

The Asnis screw system uses 6.5 mm self-tapping cannulated screws. Three screws in a triangular pattern are recommended for undisplaced or impacted intracapsular fractures. For displaced fractures four screws in a

diamond pattern are suggested. It is postulated that these patterns give rotatory stability.

An alternative system, the Ullevaal screws (7 mm in diameter) are recommended to be placed with two distal and one proximal screw. One potential disadvantage with this

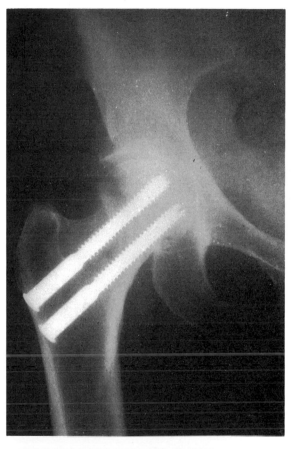

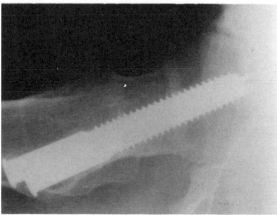

Fig. 5.11   Correct positioning of Garden screws.

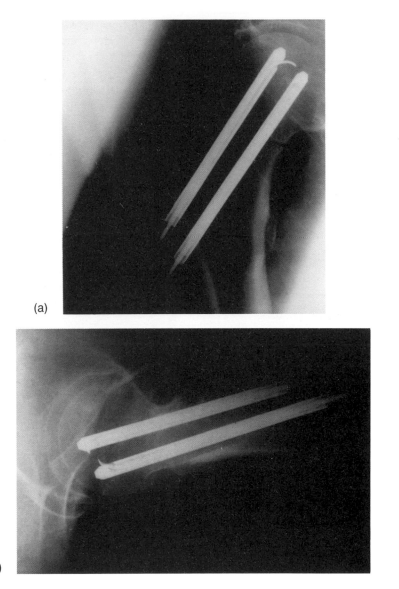

(a)

(b)

Fig. 5.12(a,b)   Examples of parallel Hansson pins.

screw positioning is that the separation of the two distal screws can damage the cortical bone of the calcar region. The risk is usually greatest on the dorsal side, where the screw may lie partly outside the femoral neck and then re-enter the head.

Knowles's pins are thinner and may be used in larger numbers. They are mainly used for children's fractures or slipped upper femoral epiphysis. Deyerle pins are positioned through a plate at the lateral side of the

trochanter. The Deyerle technique demands a larger exposure of the lateral part of the femur and longer operation times to place multiple pins. An unacceptably high risk of penetration of pins into the acetabulum has been reported.

The surgical technique for a three- or four-screw fixation is similar to that for two screws. Under X-ray control guidewires are placed across the fracture site and passed up to the subchondral region. Figure 5.13 illustrates

Correct positioning of three screws

Distal screw entry point in lateral cortex level with the middle or lower part of the lesser trochanter

Distal screw lying just superior to the calcar on the anteroposterior (AP) radiograph

Distal screw lying centrally on the lateral radiograph

Proximal screws within the centre of the femoral head on the AP radiograph

One of the proximal screws posteriorly positioned on the lateral X-ray to obtain cortical bone 67All screws should engage a separate part of the femoral head and not be touching

Tip of both screws about 5 mm from the joint line

what the authors believe is correct positioning of three screws. Note the cortical bone contact of the lower screw on the AP view and the posterior cortical contact on the lateral view. The surgeon should try to ensure that each screw is placed in a separate area of the femoral head. The tip of the screws should be about 5 mm from the joint line, to obtain a good grip on the stronger subchondral bone.

Measurement of the correct screw length is made using a depth gauge. This may require an addition of 5 mm to allow for the screw head, depending on the system used.

Dynamic hip screw fixation

A screw plate of the same type as used for trochanteric fractures (dynamic hip screw, Ambi or compression hip screws) has been used for femoral neck fractures, with a shorter two-hole plate (Fig. 5.14).

The surgical technique for insertion of the implant is the same as that described in Chapter 6, with the following additional points:

1 The lateral femoral cortex needs to be exposed via a 6–10 cm lateral skin incision, as described in Chapter 6.
2 The lag screw is positioned in the middle third of the femoral head in both the AP and lateral views.
3 The tip of the lag screw should lie closer to the articular cartilage than in a trochanteric fracture. For a centrally placed lag screw the joint line to screw tip distance should be less than 5 mm.
4 Because a single large lag screw is being used there is a risk that the proximal fragment will be rotated either as the screw is inserted or in the postoperative period. Rotation during the operation may be prevented by using one or two additional guidewires passed across the fracture site. A supplementary cancellous screw has been recommended to be placed immediately superior and parallel to the dynamic hip screw lag screw, to prevent rotation in the post-operative period (Fig. 5.15). However, clinical studies have not

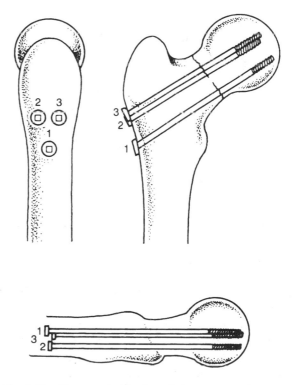

Fig. 5.13 Correct positioning of three screws.

demonstrated this additional screw to be of benefit.

5 The length of threads on the lag screw varies depending on the manufacturer. The threads should not be of a length that bridges the fracture site preventing impaction.

6 A standard angle of 135° two-hole side plate should be used. If a longer plate is used and the lag screw has not been inserted at exactly 135°, then when the plate is fixed on the femur it may produce angulation of the fracture, with the plate acting as a lever arm.

Compression of the fracture

Interoperative compression of an intracapsular fracture can be achieved using a dynamic hip screw with the compression screw applied, or alternatively with a parallel screw method and washers at the screw heads. Compression has been advocated on the theoretical grounds that it will stabilize the fracture. Clinical studies have shown the opposite, with mechanical compression of the fracture found to be detrimental.

Postoperative management

Weight-bearing

There is some controversy as to whether postoperative mobilization should be non- or partial weight-bearing, until the fracture has united. The few clinical studies that have considered this issue have not found weight-bearing to have any influence on fracture healing. Biomechanical studies have found that the forces through the hip are not reduced by using crutches to keep the injured leg off the floor. This is because the forces generated by the muscles around the hip are greater than those from gravity. Partial weight-bearing, in which the foot is put to the floor, but some weight is taken through the crutches, may nevertheless have some effect in reducing forces across the hip joint.

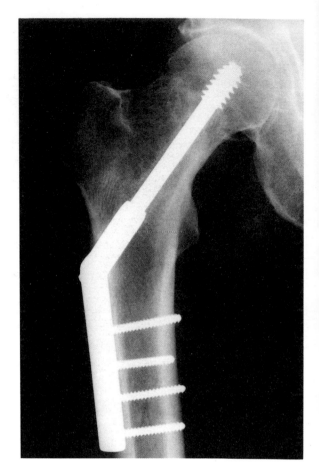

Fig. 5.14 A dynamic hip screw used for an intracapsular fracture. Conventionally a two-hole side plate will suffice and ideally the tip of the lag screw should be placed closer to the joint.

For elderly patients who will find it difficult to comply with constraints there should be no restriction on weight-bearing. For younger patients a period of partial weight-bearing until the fracture shows radiographic evidence of healing may be prudent.

Hip function

There should be no restriction on the range of hip movements. Activities such as getting in and out of a car should be permitted as soon as able. However, torsional strain under load with twisting of the leg, is best avoided until the fracture has united.

Follow-up

Normally outpatient follow-up is arranged to permit X-rays of the hip to be taken to confirm fracture union. This is essential for the younger patient because complications such as early avascular necrosis or non-union may require intervention before symptoms become apparent. It can be argued that routine radiological follow-up is not necessary for the elderly unless the hip is symptomatic. This is because further interventions will only be undertaken on those with symptomatic problems of fracture healing. This depends on whether adequate primary care is available in the community.

Complications

Internal fixation of the displaced intracapsular fracture has a higher rate of surgical complications and subsequent re-operation compared

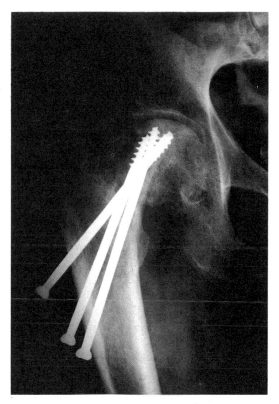

Fig. 5.16 An intracapsular fracture which was fixed with three parallel screws. The fracture has re-displaced with the lower two screws losing their hold in the femoral head.

to fixation of an undisplaced intracapsular fracture or after primary arthroplasty. The three main complications that may occur are early re-displacement, non-union or avascular necrosis. In clinical practice there is some overlap between these and it may be difficult to distinguish between early re-displacement and non-union and non-union and avascular necrosis.

Early re-displacement

This usually presents with increasing pain at the hip and recurrence of the limb deformity. It is confirmed on X-ray (Figs 5.16 and 5.17). In most cases the most appropriate option will be replacement of the femoral head. If the patient is younger than 70 years, or there is damage to the acetabulum, total hip arthroplasty should be considered. Otherwise a

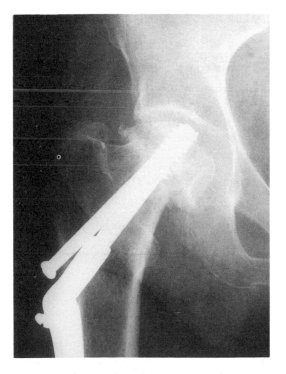

Fig. 5.15 An intracapsular fracture fixed with a dynamic hip screw and supplementary screw. Avascular necrosis of the femoral head has occurred, resulting in the tip of the lag screw penetrating into the joint.

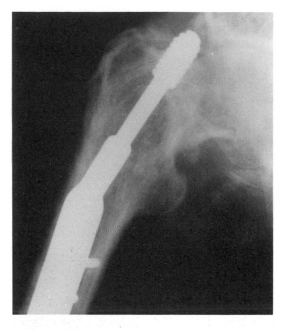

Fig. 5.17 Failure of fixation of an intracapsular fracture treated by fixation with dynamic hip screw. The implant has cut out from the femoral head.

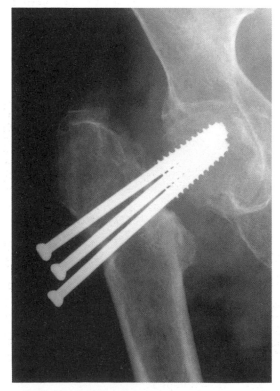

Fig. 5.18 Non-union of an intracapsular fracture fixed with three parallel cancellous screws. There has been complete re-absorption of the femoral neck.

hemiarthroplasty is the most reasonable option.

In a very young patient (probably less than 55 years), attempt to salvage the femoral head may be indicated. Open reduction, re-fixation and muscle pedicle bone grafting or femoral osteotomy is most likely to achieve successful union.

Non-union of the fracture

This usually accompanies failure of fixation with cut-out of the screws from the position of fixation. However, occasionally it develops in the presence of a stable fixation with persistence of the fracture line or even with absorption of the femoral neck (Fig. 5.18). It may present gradually or acutely with increasing pain in the hip, associated with painful movements and shortening of the leg.

Treatment may be expectant in the hope that fracture healing will eventually occur; generally, however, arthroplasty is indicated. If preservation of the femoral head is felt to be paramount, the options are either vascularized muscle pedicle bone grafting of the fracture site or osteotomy to realign the plane of the fracture to achieve compression. Such procedures are technically demanding and certainly not for the trainee.

Table 5.1 Radiographic signs of avascular necrosis

Blotchy or indistinct trabeculae

Areas of reduced and increased bone density within the femoral head (Fig. 5.19)

Apical flattening of the femoral head at the apex

Slightly separated areas of bone from the subchondral bone to form a 'rim sign' (Fig. 5.20)

Distortion of the femoral head with areas of depression bone – the 'bite sign' – which in more advanced stages leads to absorption of the femoral head (Fig. 5.21)

Loss of the hip joint space and acetabular damage

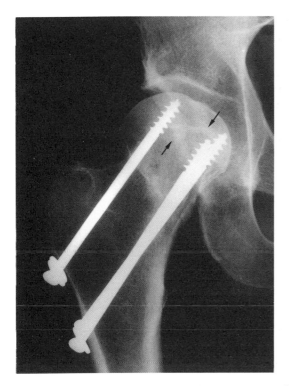

Fig. 5.19 Early avascular necrosis. There are areas of increased bone density (arrows).

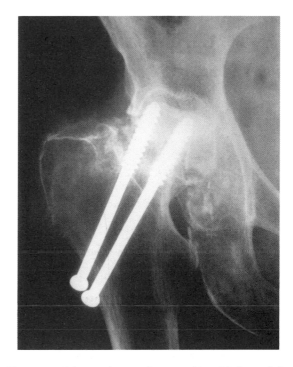

Fig. 5.21 Advanced avascular necrosis with loss of the normal shape of the femoral head from absorption. There is also damage to the acetabulum, although some of this may have been caused by the screws penetrating out of the collapsed femoral head.

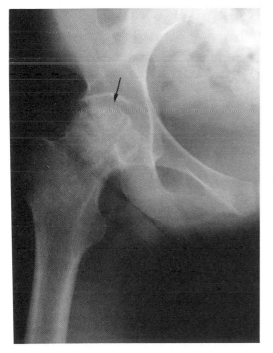

Fig. 5.20 Avascular necrosis with areas of increased and reduced density within the femoral head and a rim sign (arrow).

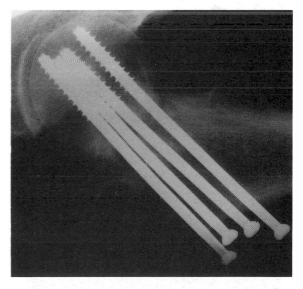

Fig. 5.22 An intracapsular fracture fixed with four cannulated cancellous screws. Collapse at the fracture site has caused increased lateral protrusion of the screw heads, which may cause discomfort.

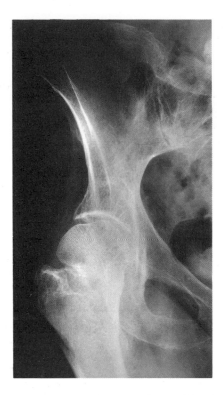
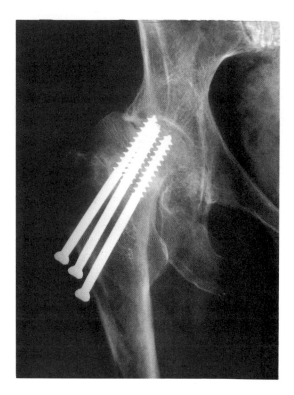

Fig. 5.23 Fragmentation of the femoral head around 6.5 mm cancellous screws.

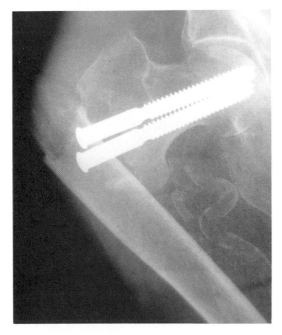

Fig. 5.24 Fracture of the femur through the insertion point of two parallel Garden screws.

Avascular necrosis

This generally occurs between 6 months and 2 years from injury and after the fracture has healed. The clinical symptoms are of increasing pain in the hip with deterioration in walking. These may pre-date the X-ray signs, which are listed in Table 5.1.

While there are techniques reported which attempt to re-vascularize the femoral head, these are only applicable where there has not been any serious collapse of the femoral head. Minor radiographic changes of the femoral head are frequently asymptomatic. For advanced necrosis the most practical option will be arthroplasty – usually total hip replacement.

Backing out of the screws

During the healing period some degree of compression in the fracture will take place. This is beneficial for the healing process, but results in about 1 cm of leg shortening. This shortening is often not noticed by the patient. At the same time there is lateral extrusion of the screw heads (Fig. 5.22). Excessive protrusion can cause discomfort when lying on the affected side, especially in thin patients. They can also give a snapping feeling with certain movements, such as rising from deep arm chairs. Treatment is by removal of the screws once the fracture is fully healed.

Other complications

These are less common and include such rare problems as fracture around the proximal ends of the screws (Fig. 5.23) or fracture around the distal end of the implant (Fig. 5.24).

Key references

Baksi DP. Treatment of post-traumatic avascular necrosis of the femoral head by multiple drilling and muscle-pedicle bone grafting. *J Bone Joint Surg* 1983; **65–B**:268–273.

Barnes R, Brown JT, Garden RS, Nicholl EA. Subcapital fractures of the femur: a prospective review. *J Bone Joint Surg* 1976; **58–B**:2–24.

Das De S, Balasubramaniam P. Anterior trochanteric muscle pedicle graft: brief report. *J Bone Joint Surg* 1991; **73–B**:171–172.

Flynn M. A new method of reduction of fractures of the neck of the femur based on anatomical studies of the hip joint. *Injury* 1974; **5**:309–317.

Graham J. Early or delayed weight-bearing after internal fixation of transcervical fracture of the femur: a clinical trial. *J Bone Joint Surg* 1968; **50–B**:562–569.

Hansson S. On the operative treatment of medial fractures of femoral neck. *Acta Orthop Scand* 1932; **3**:366–369.

Leadbetter GW. A treatment for fracture of the neck of the femur. *J Bone Joint Surg* 1933; **15**:931–941.

Meyers MH, Harvey JP, Moore TM. The muscle pedicle bone graft in the treatment of displaced fracture of the femoral neck: indications, operative technique, and results. *Orthop Clin North Am* 1974; **5**:779–792.

Parker MJ, Pryor GA. *Hip Fracture Management.* Blackwell Scientific Publications, Oxford, 1993.

Smith-Petersen MN. Approach to and exposure of the hip joint for mold arthroplasty. *J Bone Surg* 1949; **31–A**:40.

Smith-Petersen MN, Cave EF, Van Gorder GW. Intracapsular fractures of the neck of the femur. Treatment of internal fixation. *Arch Swg* 1931; **23**:715–759.

Strömqvist B, Nilsson LT, Thorngren K-G. Femoral neck fracture fixation with hook-pins: 2-year results and learning curve in 626 prospective cases. *Acta Orthop Scand* 1992; **63**:282–287.

Tronzo RG. Hip nails for all occasions. *Orthop Clin North Am* 1974; **5**:479–491.

6

Extramedullary fixation of extracapsular fractures

The extramedullary fixation of an extracapsular fracture entails applying a plate to the lateral surface of the proximal femur, connected to a pin or screw placed within the femoral head and neck. As discussed in Chapter 2, this method of treatment is recommended for most trochanteric hip fractures and high subtrochanteric fractures (Fig. 6.1). The dynamic hip screw (DHS) should be regarded as the implant of choice.

Surgical technique

Chapter 4 refers to the positioning of the patient on the fracture table. Fracture reduction and subsequent positioning of the implant must be checked by the X-ray image intensifier.

Reduction of the fracture

Undisplaced fractures can be fixed without any reduction. However, this must be carefully confirmed, as what may appear to be an undisplaced fracture can actually be displaced into slight varus (Fig. 6.2). Measurement of the trabecular angle will rapidly determine if any displacement has occurred.

Closed reduction

For all displaced fractures it is essential to reduce the fracture prior to fixation. To achieve maximum mechanical stability, a slight degree of valgus of the femoral neck is recommended (Fig. 6.3). A valgus reduction is advocated as this improves mechanical stability, thereby reducing the risk of fixation failure. In addition, shortening of the limb is reduced. A valgus reduction is normally easily achieved by applying longitudinal traction to the limb using the fracture table. Sufficient traction should be applied until the trabecular angle on

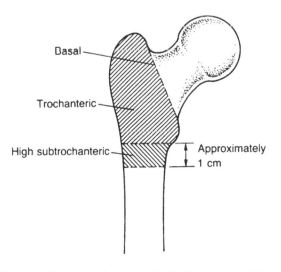

Fig. 6.1 Fractures that are suitable for extramedullary fixation.

the anteroposterior (AP) X-ray measures 165–175°.

On the lateral view it should be possible to draw a straight line to bisect the femoral head, neck and shaft (Fig. 6.4). Longitudinal traction to the limb normally results in correct alignment, but if this fails the fracture must be reduced openly.

The degree of rotation in which the foot is placed for surgery may be determined by screening the fracture, although in many cases this can be difficult to assess. As a general rule the patient's patella should face the ceiling once the leg is positioned on the fracture table. Fixation of an extracapsular fracture with more than 10° of internal rotation is not recommended as it may result in a permanent rotational deformity.

Open reduction

Failure to achieve a satisfactory closed reduction dictates that an open reduction has to be performed. Normally there is no difficulty in achieving satisfactory alignment on the AP radiograph. It is angulation of the fracture site on the lateral X-ray that must be corrected (Fig. 6.5).

Correction of angulation at the fracture site may be achieved by one or two methods. A bone clamp may be placed around the proximal femoral shaft, distal to the fracture site. The femur is then lifted upwards. Alternatively a bone lever may be placed below the fracture site and pressed superiorly (Fig. 6.6).

Once the angulation is corrected, this position should be maintained by an assistant whilst the lag screw is inserted. Alternatively the reduction may be held by guidewires passed across the fracture. Occasionally, however, especially in obese patients these wires may bend and fail to hold the reduction. Rarely the displacement on the lateral view may be so extreme that there is little bone-to-bone contact (Fig. 6.7). This must be corrected before insertion of the lag screw by similar methods described.

Only rarely is wide exposure of the fracture site required to achieve an adequate reduction.

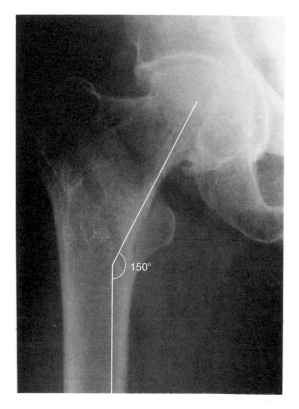

Fig. 6.2 An apparently undisplaced fracture, but the trabecular angle is 150°. The normal angle is 160°, indicating that this fracture has displaced into varus. The fracture must be reduced before fixation.

Extension dissection and exposure of the fracture site should be avoided if possible, as this causes excessive bleeding and increases the risk of sepsis and non-union.

Osteotomy

A number of osteotomies around the fracture site have been recommended in the past. They were only designed to be used with static nail plates to try and prevent the fracture collapsing. With a dynamic implant such as the DHS there are no indications for any osteotomy. A number of clinical studies have indicated that using an osteotomy with the DHS results in an increase in the operating time, operative blood loss, sepsis, fixation failure rate and mortality. There should therefore be no need to perform an osteotomy when using the DHS.

Surgical approach to the femur

With the patient positioned on the fracture table the skin is prepared and the area isolated, preferably with a plastic isolation drape (Fig. 4.8). A longitudinal incision is made from the level of the greater trochanter extending approximately 15 cm distally (Fig. 6.8). With experience, however, it is possible to limit the length of incision to that equal to the length of the plate which is to be used.

Subcutaneous fat is divided to expose the shiny layer of fascia lata. It is helpful to separate the fat off the fascia lata in the line of the incision, as this makes the fascia more readily identified when closing the wound.

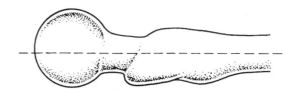

Fig. 6.4 Correct reduction on the lateral X-ray means that the femoral head, neck, trochanteric region and shaft are all in a straight line.

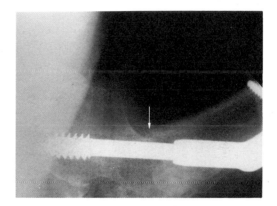

Fig. 6.5 Angulation of the fracture on the lateral X-ray must be corrected before inserting the lag screw. Fixing the fracture in a displaced position as shown here results in a mechanically unstable conformation. In addition the dynamic hip screw is forced to be placed in a posterior position because of cortical bone in the femoral neck (arrow) and this results in a high risk of fixation failure.

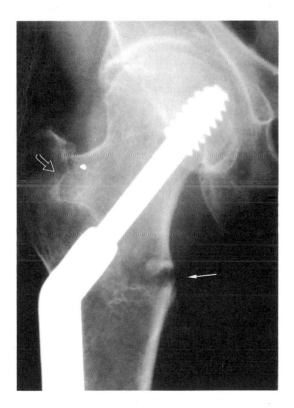

Fig. 6.3 A valgus reduction is achieved using longitudinal traction and results in an ideal trabecular angle of 170°. X-rays taken in the early postoperative period show a gap medially (arrow) created by the valgus reduction; this soon disappears with compression of the fracture and controlled collapse of the fracture with weight-bearing. Bony contact and stability are initially provided laterally (open arrow).

The fascia lata is split in the line of the skin incision (Fig. 6.9).

The vastus lateralis muscle is now exposed. Two alternative approaches are now available to the femur. For the 'Silk' approach the vastus lateralis is lifted anteriorly and the femur approached in the tissue plane between the vastus lateralis and the lateral intermuscular septum. The alternative approach is directly through the vastus lateralis muscle, splitting the muscle fibres in the line of the skin incision (Fig. 6.10).

The Silk approach has the advantage of causing less muscle damage, and on completion of the fixation the muscle falls back into place to cover the plate. Bleeding from vessels perforating the lateral intermuscular septum can be troublesome and must be controlled.

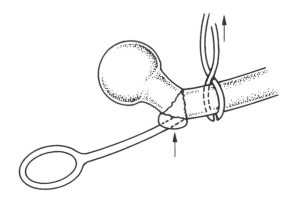

Fig. 6.6 Methods of correction of angulation on the lateral X-ray view. Either the femur is lifted superiorly by a bone clamp, or the bone at the fracture site is elevated by means of a bone lever.

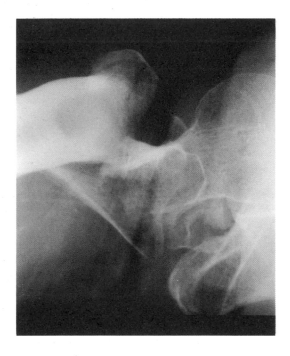

Fig. 6.7 Such extreme displacement on the lateral X-ray always requires open reduction.

The direct muscle-splitting approach can result in a greater blood loss and more muscle damage, but gives better access if a long plate is to be used.

Once the femur is reached the lateral surface of the femur is exposed using a periosteal elevator, to strip the muscle fibres of vastus lateralis off their bone attachment. Dissection

of the femur should be confined to that area of femur on which the plate will be placed.

Positioning of the guidewire

The guidewire is next positioned within the femoral head, and this then determines the position of the lag screw. Most surgeons are aware that correct positioning of the lag screw will reduce the chance of fixation failure. However, correct reduction of the fracture is the prerequisite for accurate positioning of the lag screw, as illustrated in Figure 6.11 for reduction in the AP X-ray and Figure 6.5 for reduction in the lateral view.

Placing a guidewire just anterior to the femoral neck may be useful to aid alignment (Fig. 6.12). Do not place this guidewire too far medially or anteriorly in order to avoid damage to the femoral artery. Alternatively a guidewire can be placed anterior to the leg on top of the sterile draping, to give an idea of the intended position of the guidewire on the AP view.

A guidewire is now inserted into the femoral neck and head. This is generally done by connecting the guidewire to a power drill. The 135° angle guide should be used to obtain the correct guidewire alignment with the femur (Fig. 6.13).

Generally there should be no reason to use any other than a 135° plate, although occasionally the angles of 130° and 140° may be preferred. Using a lower-angled plate increases the risk of the lag screw jamming and using an angle of greater than 140° results in superior screw placement which is unacceptable.

In many cases accurate positioning of the guidewire is made easier by inserting a guidewire in a slightly superior position in the femoral neck. The position of the guidewire is then studied on the AP and lateral radiographs. A 3.2 mm drill or awl is then used to make a hole in the lateral femoral cortex at the estimated site of insertion of a second guidewire, immediately inferior to the first guidewire (Fig. 6.14). The second guidewire mounted on a Jacob's chuck may then be

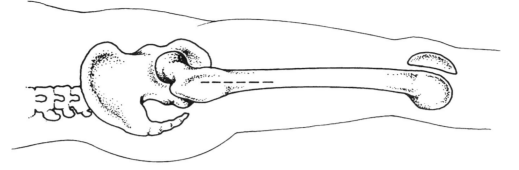

Fig. 6.8 The skin extends distally from the greater trochanter. The incision will need to be longer if a long plate or open reduction of the fracture is indicated.

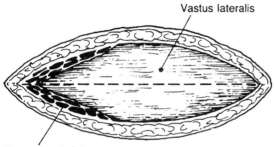

Vastus lateralis

Tensor fascia latae

Fig. 6.9 The fascia lata is exposed and then divided in the line of the skin incision.

inserted by hand in a careful manner, checking its position on the AP and lateral radiographs as it is inserted.

An alternative technique is to place an awl on the lateral femoral cortex and carefully check its position on the AP and lateral radiographs, aiming at the desired position for the lag screw in the femoral head using a guidewire held anterior to the femur. The awl is used to perforate the lateral femoral cortex, allowing a guidewire to be inserted through this entry point.

This technique allows an accurate and controlled insertion of the guidewire. It is important to spend time at this stage ensuring that the guidewire comes to lie in the correct position, that is, an inferior/central position on the AP view and central on the lateral view (Fig. 6.13).

Placing the guidewire at exactly 135° to the femoral shaft is preferable, especially for undisplaced and subtrochanteric fractures (see Fig. 6.30). For an unstable displaced fracture there is a degree of tolerance, as the instability of the fracture will correct for small differences in the angle. If, however, there is a large difference in the angle from the optimum of 135° once the plate is applied, the proximal fragment may be forced into a position of excessive valgus or varus angulation.

It is essential to position the guidewire accurately within the femoral head as this will reduce the risk of fixation failure (Fig. 6.15). All clinical studies indicate that the lag screw should be placed centrally or slightly inferior on the AP X-ray and centrally on the lateral X-ray. A few surgeons have previously recommended a slightly posterior screw position on the lateral X-ray. This is incorrect, as all clinical studies have indicated that a central position is best. Superior, posterior or anterior screw positioning of the lag screw should never be accepted.

Fracture reduction and screw positioning are the two main factors which will influence the success of fixation. Table 6.1 gives the approximate risks of fixation failure depending on the degree of fracture reduction and screw positioning.

For most extracapsular fractures the guidewire is inserted through an intact lateral femoral cortex. There are however occasions when the fracture involves this area of femoral cortex and the guidewire will then be inserted directly into the fracture site (see Fig. 6.35). Extreme care needs to be taken with this type of fracture as the lateral cortical comminution causes severe instability and a higher risk of

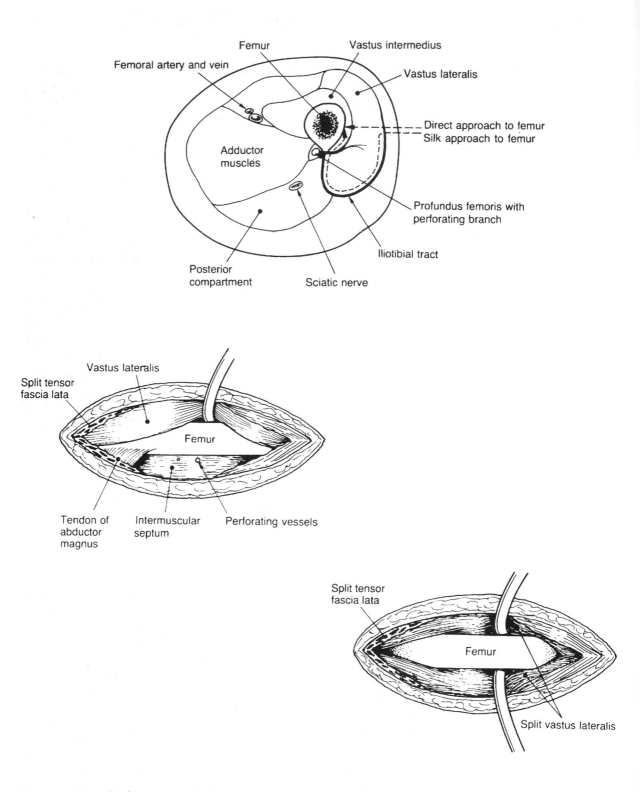

Fig. 6.10 Once the fascia lata is divided the femur may be approached either by lifting the muscle anteriorly, or directly through the muscle.

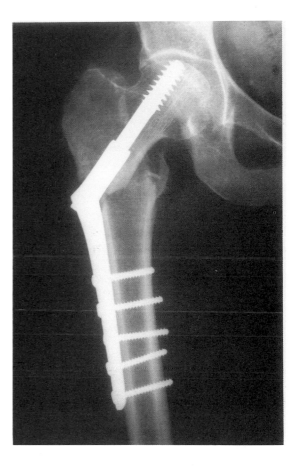

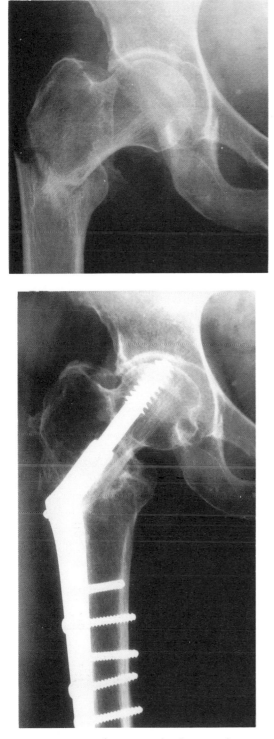

Fig. 6.11 Incorrect fracture reduction on the antero-posterior view. Post-operative trabecular angle of 140° results in a superiorly placed screw, which has an increased risk of cutting-out of the femoral head, as demonstrated on the follow-up film.

fixation failure. This specific type of fracture is discussed in greater detail later.

Insertion of the lag screw

Having achieved the correct positioning of the guidewire, the length of the lag screw is determined. This is best achieved with a measuring gauge (Fig. 6.16). Care must be taken if the guidewire has been inserted directly into the fracture site, as the measuring gauge may also be pushed into the fracture site and give a false reading.

The lag screw should normally be placed 5–10 mm from the hip joint. This distance should be subtracted from the reading of the measuring gauge, to give the size of lag screw to be used. This measurement is also that to which the cannulated triple reamer is set,

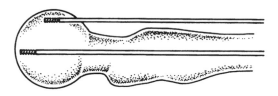

Fig. 6.12 A guidewire placed immediately anterior to the femoral neck is useful as a preliminary aid to inserting the guidewire into the femoral neck.

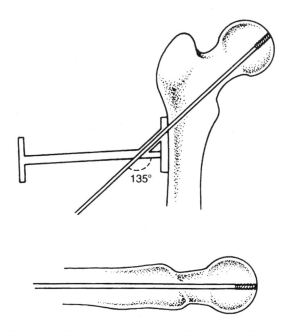

Fig. 6.13 The guidewire is inserted with the 135° angle guide. The tip of the guidewire should engage subchondral bone.

although it is best to subtract a full 10 mm for the reamer to reduce the risk of inadvertent joint penetration of the reamer. The proximal femur can now be reamed (Fig. 6.17). Whilst the larger outer barrel of the triple reamer should prevent the reamer being inserted too far medially, it is always advisable to screen the reamer with the image intensifier as it approaches the subchondral bone, to avoid inadvertent joint penetration. This is particularly important if there is comminution of the lateral femoral cortex at the site of guidewire insertion. Also check on the X-ray that the guidewire is not being pushed into the pelvis with reaming, as can occur if the wire has been bent.

Occasionally the guidewire will be pulled out of the femur on removing the reamer. In this situation it is essential to replace the guidewire and check its position on AP and lateral radiographs before continuing. The method shown in Figure 6.18 assists in accurate re-insertion of the guidewire.

The use of a tap to cut threads for the lag screw is only required in young patients with hard cancellous bone. Care needs to be taken with tapping the bone not to penetrate the femoral head with the tap and thereby damage the articular surfaces of the joint.

Next the lag screw is inserted using its introducer and the position checked on both AP and lateral X-rays (Fig. 6.19). Points to note are that the lag screw should be inserted to 5–10 mm from the joint surface. This is because the subchondral bone in this area is strong and thus this reduces the risk of lag screw migration within the femoral head. The lag screw will have one or two flat surfaces which match those on the barrel of the DHS; this prevents the lag screw turning once the plate is applied. These flat surfaces must be

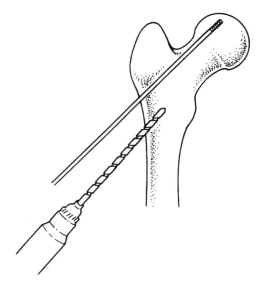

Fig. 6.14 Accurate guidewire positioning may be helped by placing a preliminary guidewire in the femoral neck in a superior position. A 3.2 mm drill hole of the lateral femoral cortex is then made immediately inferior to this, through which the final guidewire is inserted by hand.

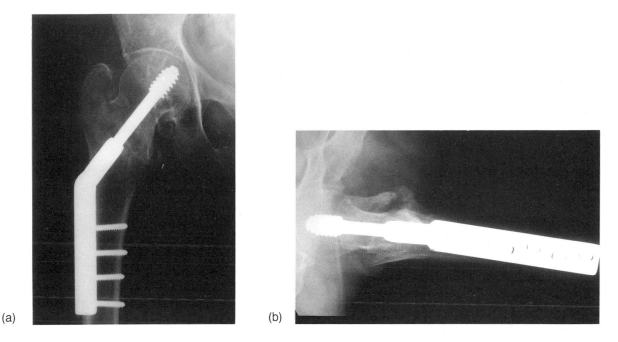

(a)   (b)

Fig. 6.15 Correct reduction and fixation of a trochanteric fracture. (a) On the anteroposterior radiograph the trabecular angle is 170° and the screw centrally placed. (b) On the lateral X-ray the lag screw is centrally placed and it is possible to draw a straight line to bisect the femoral head, neck and shaft.

correctly oriented to allow the barrel to fit; this is achieved by having the handle of the insertion device parallel to the shaft of the femur.

Application of the side plate

Following lag screw insertion the side plate is slotted on to the lag screw and gently hammered into place (Fig. 6.20). The plate must lie along the lateral surface of the femur and is held in place with a bone clamp passed around the femur. Traction from the leg is now reduced and the guidewire removed.

The length of the plate will be determined by the configuration of the fracture. As a general guide, four screws or eight cortices should be fixed distal to the fracture. The majority of fractures do not extend to the proximal screw; therefore a four-hole plate will normally suffice. However, for those fractures which are more distal, or have subtrochanteric extension, a longer plate will be

Table 6.1 Risk of fixation failure depending on the degree of fracture reduction and screw position

	Risk of fixation failure
Trabecular angle less than 160°	28%
Trabecular angle 160° or more	5%
Superior screw position	52%
Anterior screw position	55%
Posterior screw position	21%
Inferior or central position	6%
Screw correctly placed on both views*	3%

* Central or inferior on anteroposterior and central on lateral X-ray.

required (see Fig. 6.40). Preoperative planning with transparent plastic templates may be useful to determine the correct plate length.

The plate is next fixed to the femur with cortical screws (Fig. 6.21). When drilling and tapping the femur for these screws, care is

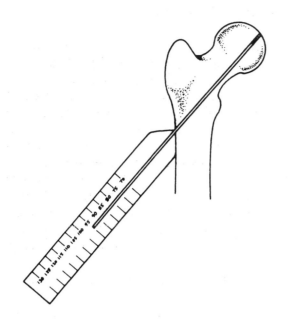

Fig. 6.16 The length of the lag screw is determined by subtracting 5–10 mm from the reading on the measuring gauge. Note that the guidewire tip is at the hip joint.

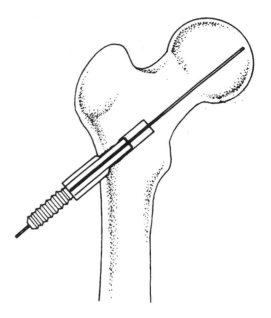

Fig. 6.18 A reversed lag screw and centring sleeve may be used to help guidewire reinsertion.

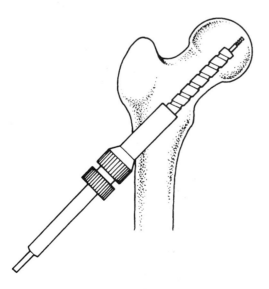

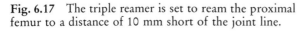

Fig. 6.17 The triple reamer is set to ream the proximal femur to a distance of 10 mm short of the joint line.

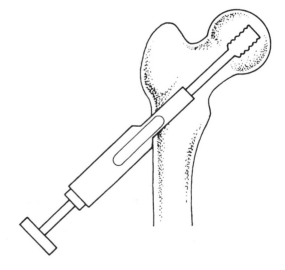

Fig. 6.19 The lag screw is inserted to a distance of 5–10 mm from the joint. The handle of the insertion device must be parallel to the femur to allow the flat surfaces of the lag screw to engage with those of the dynamic hip screw plate.

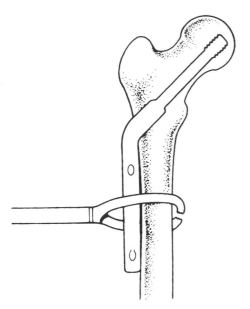

Fig. 6.20 A side plate of appropriate length is gently hammered into place and held in position with a bone clamp. It is important to ensure that the plate lies parallel to the femur.

needed not to push the drill too deeply, risking damage to the profundus femoris vessels (Fig. 6.22).

For the majority of fractures no further fixation is required and the wound can be closed. The rules of fixation given here should be satisfied.

Criteria for successful fixation

Fracture is reduced to a trabecular angle of 165–175° on the anteroposterior (AP) radiograph

Fracture is reduced on the lateral X-ray such that the femoral head, neck, trochanteric area and femoral shaft are in a straight line

Lag screw is centrally or inferiorly placed on the AP X-ray

Lag screw is centrally placed on the lateral X-ray

Lag screw tip 5–10 mm from the hip joint

Plate of sufficient length to have at least four screws (eight cortices) placed distal to the fracture

---

Closure of the wound

Irrigation of the tissues with sterile saline is recommended to remove any blood clots and tissue debris, which may act as a potential source of sepsis. Haemostasis is checked before wound closure. If vastus lateralis has been lifted anteriorly, this is allowed to fall down to cover the plate. If the surgical exposure has been extensive, the tendinous part of the vastus lateralis at the level of the greater trochanter should be repaired with an absorbable suture. If vastus lateralis has been split by the direct approach, then loose interrupted sutures should be used to close the split (Fig. 6.23).

Next fascia lata is repaired with a strong absorbable suture (Fig. 6.24).

A fat stitch is not normally required, except in the obese. The skin should be closed with an absorbable subcuticular suture (Fig. 6.25). Interrupted sutures act as a potential tract for the entry of bacteria into the wound and should be avoided. Careful and accurate opposition of skin edges is important to ensure rapid wound healing, reducing the risk of organisms entering the wound. In these

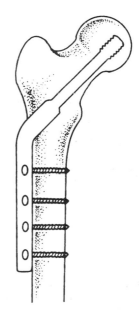

Fig. 6.21 The plate is fixed to the femur with cortical screws.

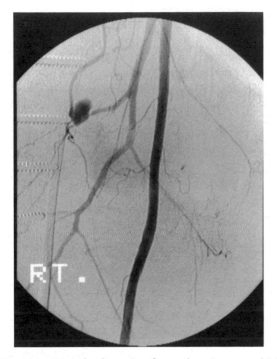

Fig. 6.22   Digital subtraction femoral angiogram which demonstrates a pseudoaneurysm of the first perforating branch of the profundus femoris artery. The aneurysm was caused during either drilling of the femur or insertion of the cortical screw. From Hanna GB, Holdsworth RJ, McCollum PT. Profunda femoris artery pseudoaneurysm following orthopaedic procedures. *Injury* 1994 **25**:477–478, with permission.

patients there is a high risk of wound contamination by urine and faeces.

Additional technical points

The versatility of the DHS allows for a number of different options regarding fracture fixation. These alternatives include the following choices.

Use of the compression screw

The compression screw is inserted into the lag screw after the plate is fixed to the femur. It may be used to compress the fracture site. Routine use of this screw is not recommended, as there is no evidence that fracture compression is beneficial. In fact it may be detrimental, especially if the compression

screw is over-tightened, as the lag screw can be pulled laterally. In addition, with fracture collapse the compression screw may protrude laterally, causing pain, or even migrate within the leg.

Use of a short barrel plate

The shorter the length of the lag screw, the less the amount of available slide. If an 80 mm lag screw is used with a standard 38 mm barrel,

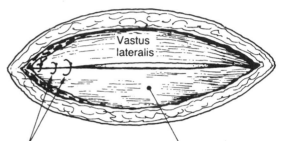

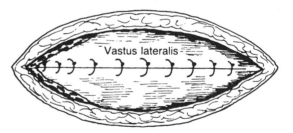

Fig. 6.23   The proximal tendinous insertion of vastus lateralis may need to be repaired if vastus lateralis was lifted superiorly. If a direct approach was used the muscle edges are approximated with absorbable interrupted sutures.

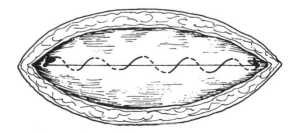

Fig. 6.24   The longitudinal incision of tensor fascia lata is closed.

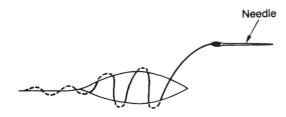

Fig. 6.25 Closure of the wound with absorbable subcuticular sutures.

there will be only 15 mm of available slide. If the lag screw runs out of slide before the fracture is healed, there will be an increased risk of cut-out of the lag screw from the femoral head. A 25 mm short barrel plate will increase the amount of available slide by 13 mm.

A short barrel plate should only be used with lag screws of 80 mm or less. For the longer lengths of lag screw there will be sufficient slide available. Furthermore there is an increased risk of lag screw jamming if a long lag screw is used with a short barrel plate.

Another potential hazard of a short barrel plate is separation of the plate from the lag screw. This can be prevented by using the compression screw (Fig. 6.26). Care needs to be taken not to over-tighten this locking screw as it may pull the lag screw laterally out of the femoral head.

Supplementary fixation

For the majority of extracapsular fractures additional fixation is not recommended as it contributes little to increased stability, prolongs surgery and increases the risk of sepsis. Inexperienced surgeons sometimes try to fix a displaced lesser trochanter fragment; such attempts may be detrimental as extensive dissection is required, with the risk of damaging surrounding structures. Furthermore, the lesser trochanter fragment in the elderly will be too weak to obtain any substantial fixation.

On occasions, however, an additional screw may be of use with subtrochanteric fracture to assist in maintaining fracture reduction, whilst

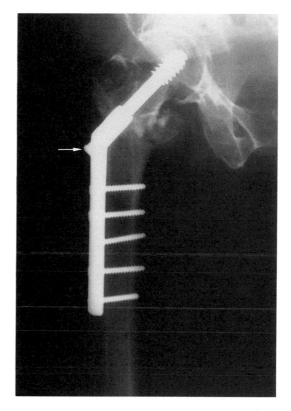

Fig. 6.26 A short barrel plate used with a 75 mm lag screw to increase the amount of available slide. Note that a compression screw has been used (arrow), not to compress the fracture but to prevent the lag screw becoming detached from the plate.

the DHS is inserted (see Fig. 6.41). This may be particularly relevant when a large medial fragment is present.

A single supplementary screw placed superior to the lag screw has been advocated to prevent rotation of the proximal fragment, which can occur if there is little soft-tissue attachment. It is however debatable if such a supplementary screw is of value and if it is not placed parallel to the lag screw it may impede collapse of the fracture.

Cerclage wires and bands are rarely of value. They may occasionally be passed around the femur to encircle a large medial fragment but it remains unproven as to what extent this increases the strength of the fixation. If wires are used, care needs to be taken to ensure that they do not prevent sliding of the lag screw.

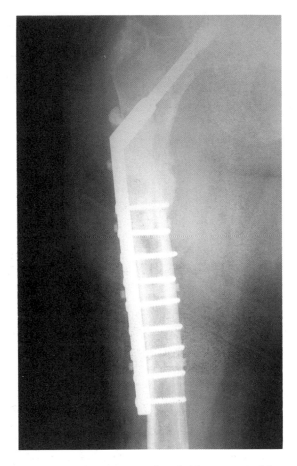

Fig. 6.27 Bone cement used to bridge a cortical bone defect in a pathological subtrochanteric fracture.

Cement augmentation

The use of bone cement, placed around the fracture site, was originally reported to produce good results. However long-term follow-up of these patients revealed a high incidence of long-term complications with fixation failure and avascular necrosis of the femoral head. Routine use of cement cannot therefore be recommended. There may be occasional indications in pathological fracture where there is extensive bone loss and limited life expectancy (Fig. 6.27).

Bone grafting

There is no evidence that bone grafting to the fracture site is necessary for acute hip fracture surgery. Grafting may even be detrimental as it prolongs surgery and may result in increased morbidity and mortality.

Use of trochanteric stabilizing plate

This is a plate which clips to the side of the DHS. It provides additional support for the greater trochanter (Fig. 6.28). The plate may be useful for those fractures in which there is extensive comminution of the lateral femoral cortex, or transverse fractures at the level of the lesser trochanter. For these fractures there is a tendency for the femur to displace medially, which reduces the area of bone-to-bone contact at the fracture site. A trochanteric stabilizing plate will prevent this medialization of the femur.

Medoff sliding plate

This is a more recently developed modification to the DHS. It consists of two interlocking side plates which allow compression

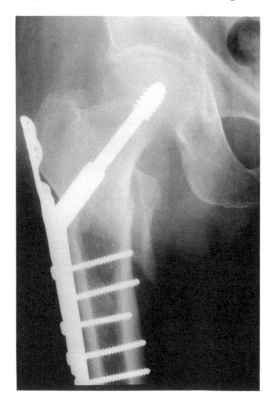

Fig. 6.28 A trochanteric stabilizing plate prevents femoral medialization and may improve fracture stability in selected fractures.

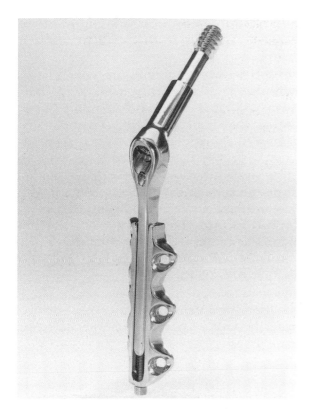

Fig. 6.29 The Medoff sliding plate.

to occur longitudinally along the line of the femur as well as along the line of the lag screw (Fig. 6.29) The implant also has the capability of allowing longitudinal interoperative compression and locking of sliding along the lag screw.

The possible advantages of this plate are currently being studied, but it may be valuable in fractures within the area of bone just below the level of the lesser trochanter. For these fractures the Medoff plate allows dynamic compression to occur across the fracture site. Many of these fractures, if fixed with a standard DHS, would result in a static fixation. Such an example is illustrated in Figure 6.38.

Specific fracture types

Extracapsular fractures vary in severity from a simple undisplaced two-part fracture to an extensively comminuted fracture. In addition the configuration of the fracture line and the

anatomical site of the fracture need to be considered. As discussed in Chapter 2, no method of fracture classification will comprehensively describe all these features. However, it is important to recognize the specific fracture types discussed below.

Undisplaced fractures

These fractures may be missed at diagnosis as the radiographic signs may not be readily apparent. This type of fracture may be treated conservatively; however, operative treatment is recommended to enable unrestricted and immediate mobilization, with a reduced risk of fracture displacement occurring.

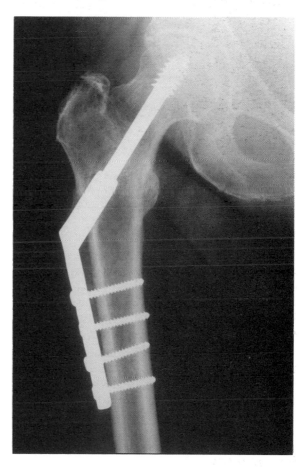

Fig. 6.30 An undisplaced trochanteric fracture fixed with a dynamic hip screw. The lag screw was not inserted at exactly 135° and therefore the plate is not parallel to the femur.

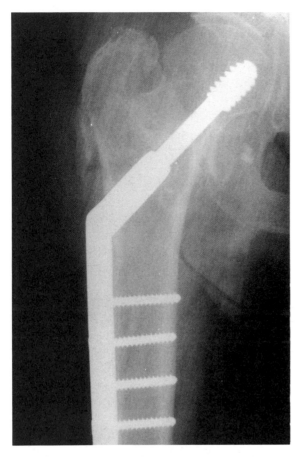

Fig. 6.31 A basal fracture fixed with the dynamic hip screw.

Surgical treatment of this type of fracture with a DHS is relatively straightforward, with a low risk of fixation failure. No fracture reduction is required. The only technical point of note is that the guidewire should be inserted at exactly 135°. Failure to achieve this means that the plate will not lie comfortably against the femur (Fig. 6.30).

Basal fracture

This refers to a two-part fracture with the fracture line running along the intertrochanteric line (Fig. 6.31). Some fracture classification systems consider a basal fracture as an intracapsular fracture, but it is best considered an extracapsular fracture, as the treatment and prognosis are akin to that of a trochanteric fracture.

Displaced basal fractures are reduced to a slight degree of valgus by longitudinal traction. Only rarely is open reduction required for this type of fracture. The soft tissue attachments to the proximal fragment may be insufficient to prevent rotation of the femoral head on lag screw insertion (Fig. 6.32). Rotation of the proximal fragment may be seen on screening the fracture during insertion of the lag screw, or by placing a finger along the anterior femoral neck and feeling for rotation.

Rotation of the proximal head fragment may be prevented by using a supplementary guidewire, placed superior to the lag screw. An alternative method is to resist rotation manually with a finger placed anterior to the femoral neck.

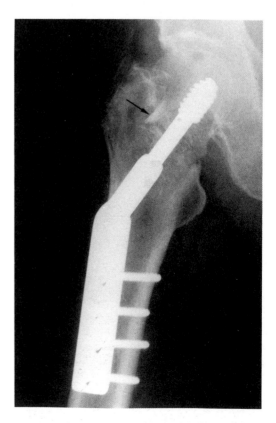

Fig. 6.32 A basal fracture fixed with the dynamic hip screw. Rotation of the proximal fragment occurred so the calcar was lying superiorly (arrow).

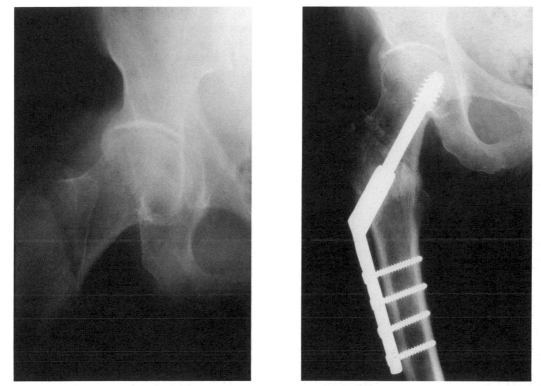

Fig. 6.33   A displaced two-part trochanteric fracture fixed with a dynamic hip screw.

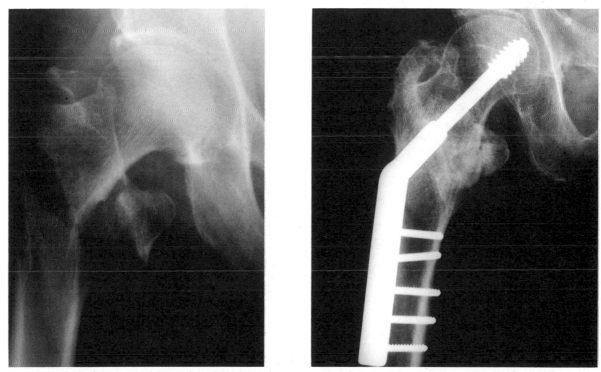

Fig. 6.34   A comminuted displaced trochanteric fracture correctly fixed with a dynamic hip screw.

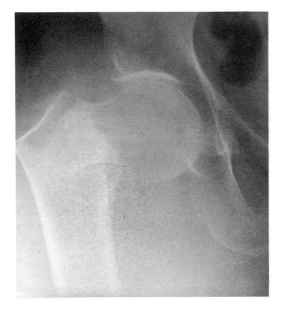

Fig. 6.35 A trochanteric fracture with comminution of the lateral femoral cortex. The key feature to note is the extensive comminution of the lateral femoral cortex at the site of lag screw inversion.

Displaced two-part trochanteric fractures

This type of fracture has a low incidence of fixation failure. The fracture is easily reduced to an anatomical or slight valgus position with longitudinal traction (Fig. 6.33).

Displaced and comminuted trochanteric fractures

This is the most frequently encountered type of trochanteric fracture. Reduction of the fracture to a valgus position is recommended and generally easily achieved by longitudinal traction (Fig. 6.34). With correct reduction and implant positioning, fixation failure should be infrequent.

Trochanteric fracture with comminution of the lateral femoral cortex

This fracture type is less common, but it is important to recognize its characteristics pre-operatively as there will frequently be technical problems of fixation and an increased risk of fixation failure. On the AP radiograph

there will be a short horizontal proximal fragment, with extensive comminution of the lateral femoral cortex, and the femoral shaft may be displaced medially. The lesser trochanter may or may not be included in the fracture (Fig. 6.35). On the lateral radiograph there is invariably displacement with angulation at the fracture site.

Direct insertion of the lag screw into the fracture site may be utilized in reducing the fracture. A valgus position may be achieved by using the insertion handle and manually reducing the fracture. In addition, reduction of the fracture on the lateral view may be achieved by a similar method. Correct reduction and central lag screw positioning are critical for this type of fracture, to reduce the chance of fixation failure.

Due to the extensive comminution of the

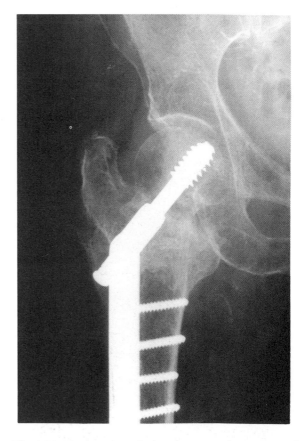

Fig. 6.36 A short barrel plate increases the amount of lag screw slide. Note that a compression screw was used to prevent lag screw separation from the short barrel, not to compress the fracture.

lateral femoral cortex, the guidewire and lag screw will be inserted directly into the proximal fragment. Because of this the lag screw invariably measures 70–80 mm in length. Once the plate is applied to the femur there is no bony support to prevent the femoral shaft displacing medially, further reducing the amount of available slide for the lag screw.

This combination of a short lag screw with femoral medialization results in early utilization of lag screw slide. In this situation if the lag screw is well-placed within the femoral head, then there is an increased risk of the plate detaching from the femur, whilst if the lag screw has been inappropriately placed within the femoral head, there is a high risk of cut-out.

In order to reduce the chances of fixation failure, modifications to the normal fixation devices have been advocated. Figure 6.36 illustrates a short barrel plate, which increases the amount of available lag screw slide. Figure 6.28 shows a trochanteric stabilizing plate which can be used to prevent femoral medialization by abutting against the remains of the greater trochanter.

Trochanteric fracture with subtrochanteric extension

In approximately 5% of trochanteric fractures there will be extension of the fracture line distally into the subtrochanteric region and even to the femoral diaphysis (Fig. 6.37). Such fractures may be treated using an intramedullary nail, but for the majority the DHS will suffice, provided a plate of sufficient length is chosen. A plate of sufficient length to allow a minimum of eight cortices fixed distal to the fracture should be used.

Reversed fracture line

The fracture line of a typical trochanteric fracture runs obliquely in an inferior-medial

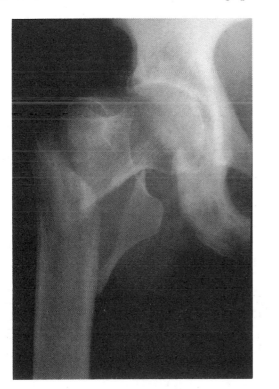
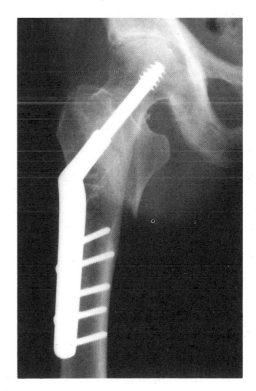

Fig. 6.37 A trochanteric fracture with a subtrochanteric extension extending to the level of the uppermost cortical screw. The pelvis shows changes of Paget's disease which probably also involved the fracture site and caused the increased blood loss which necessitated the use of a suction drain at the time of surgery.

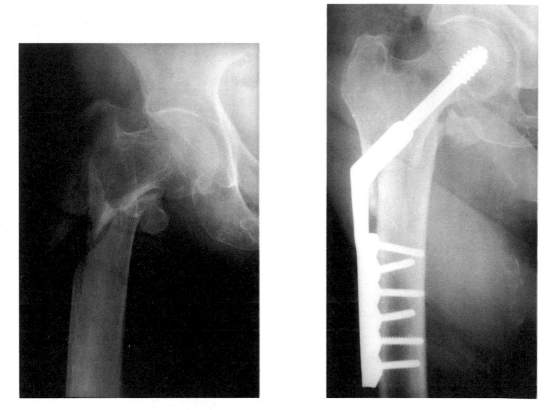

Fig. 6.38   A reversed fracture line. The adductor muscles tend to pull the distal fragment medially. The fracture was fixed with a Medoff modification of a DHS, which allows longitudinal compression to occur along the line of the femur. Had the fracture been fixed with a standard DHS, the intact lateral femoral cortical bone in the proximal fragment below the site of lag screw insertion would prevent any compression occurring along the fracture site.

direction from the greater to the lesser trochanter. A fracture running in the opposite direction is referred to as a reversed fracture line (Fig. 6.38). The forces acting across this fracture are different, with a tendency for the distal fragment to be pulled medially due to force of the adductor muscles. Theoretically, this type of fracture may require a longer length of plate to reduce the risk of fixation failure. A trochanteric stabilizing plate would prevent femoral medialization or alternatively a Medoff plate may be opportune. Intramedullary fixation is an alternative method of fixation.

'High' subtrochanteric fracture

The division between a high and low subtrochanteric fracture depends on whether, if a

DHS were used it would act as a dynamic or static implant (Fig. 6.39). With a dynamic fixation, continuous compression across the fracture site is achieved. For a static fixation then the fracture configuration prevents any collapse occurring at the fracture site.

The DHS is recommended as the treatment of choice for high subtrochanteric fractures. The principles of fixation are the same as that described previously, that is, a valgus reduction and central positioning of the lag screw. A five or six-hole side plate is normally sufficient for eight femoral cortices to be securely fixed (Fig. 6.40).

'Low' subtrochanteric fracture

If a DHS is used to fix a low subtrochanteric fracture, then it will act as a static implant.

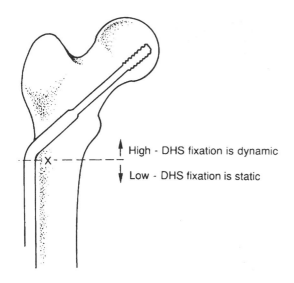

↑ High - DHS fixation is dynamic

↓ Low - DHS fixation is static

Fig. 6.39 High and low subtrochanteric fractures. The distinction is made by the area of bone (X). A fracture distal to this point cannot collapse and compress along the line of the lag screw.

Table 6.2 Differences between dynamic and static hip fracture fixation

	Dynamic	Static
Recommended fracture reduction	Valgus	Anatomical
Operative fracture compression	Not recommended	Recommended
Postoperative fracture collapse	Occurs	Prevented
Risk of non-union	Very low	Increased

Such a fixation has a higher risk of delayed union and non-union, with a resultant increased incidence of fixation failure. In addition, because of the more distal site of the fracture, a longer DHS plate of 8–10 holes is required to achieve a stable fixation. Surgery to insert such a long plate is inevitably more prolonged, with greater blood loss. Because of these factors, low subtrochanteric fractures are probably better treated with an intramedullary fixation device.

If a DHS is used for this type of fracture, the surgical principles differ considerably from those of a dynamic fixation (Table 6.2). Because postoperative fracture collapse is not possible, it is imperative that no gap exists at the fracture site. In order to achieve this the fractures should be reduced to an anatomical position. Reduction to a valgus position leaves a gap at the medial cortex which will not be closed by fracture collapse, as may occur with a dynamic fixation.

If the DHS is used to fix such a fracture (Fig. 6.41), the guidewire and lag screw must be inserted at exactly 135°. Failure to achieve this will result in a gap appearing at the fracture site either medially or laterally as the plate is fixed to the femur (Fig. 6.42). Extensive exposure of the femur is generally

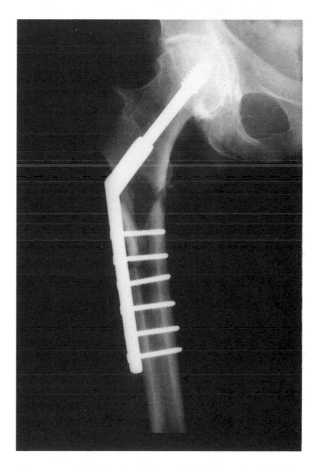

Fig. 6.40 A high subtrochanteric fracture fixed with a six-hole dynamic hip screw plate.

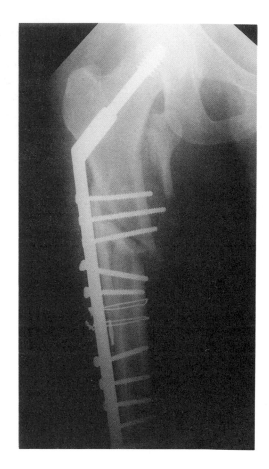

Fig. 6.42 The dynamic hip screw was not inserted at exactly 135° for this 'low' subtrochanteric fracture. This resulted in a gap at the medial fracture side, which in this static fixation cannot be closed by collapse at the fracture site.

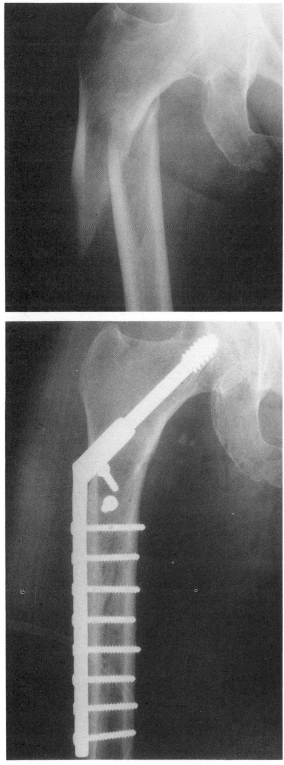

Fig. 6.41 Good dynamic hip screw fixation of a 'low' subtrochanteric fracture. Interfragmentary screws have been used to hold the fracture reduced.

required, with the possibility of high blood loss.

Postoperative management

The DHS is designed as a load-bearing implant and therefore following surgery all patients should be mobilized and full weight-bearing allowed. There need be no restriction on hip movement. If a drain has been used, then this should not be retained for more than 48 hours after surgery. Blood loss from a trochanteric fracture is often in excess of 1 litre and blood transfusion is frequently required. The haemoglobin should therefore be checked on the day following surgery.

Pain in the hip, thigh or even knee region is frequently prolonged after an extracapsular fracture and the patient may need regular analgesics in the first 1–3 months from injury until the fracture unites. This persistent pain is one of the reasons why a patient with an extracapsular fracture may take more time to recover mobility than those patients with an intracapsular fracture. Outpatient follow-up at 4–6 weeks from surgery may be arranged to permit X-rays of the hip to be taken to confirm fracture union is occurring without any adverse complications.

Complications of DHS fixation

Cut-out

The DHS is a very forgiving implant, but its main complication is cut-out of the screw

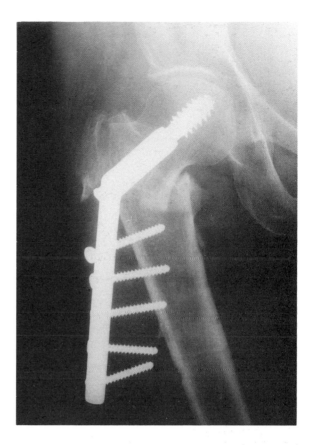

Fig. 6.44 Detachment of the plate from the femur. Note that the lag screw was inserted directly into the fracture site but a long barrel plate was used. The dynamic hip screw ran out of slide before fracture consolidation had occurred. Had the lag screw not been well-placed, cut-out would have occurred. The use of a short barrel plate may have prevented this complication.

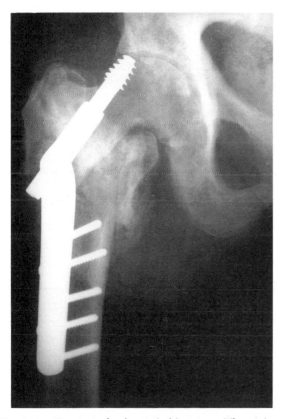

Fig. 6.43 Cut-out of a dynamic hip screw. The patient has Paget's disease of the femur which delays fracture union and increases the risk of cut-out.

from the femoral head. This occurs in approximately 2–10% of cases, but the incidence is strongly related to the quality of the surgery performed. Cut-out can be recognized clinically by increasing pain and a recurrence of the shortening and external rotation deformity seen preoperatively. However, these signs can be misleading; there may often be prolonged pain after extracapsular fracture. Furthermore, if the lesser trochanter has been avulsed, the leg will often remain externally rotated. The diagnosis can usually be made easily by X-ray (Fig. 6.43), although a good lateral view may be required, if the cut-out is not clearly apparent on the AP view.

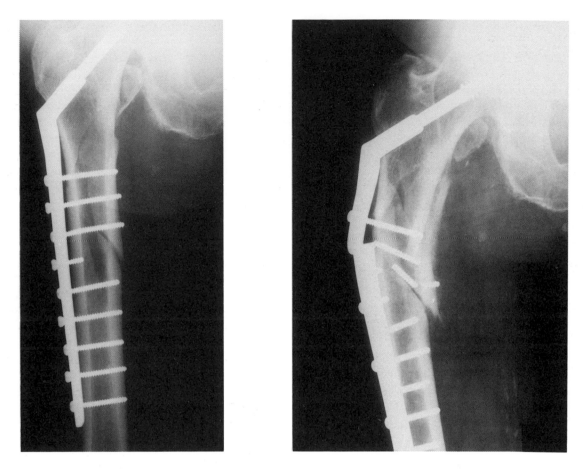

Fig. 6.45 A comminuted low subtrochanteric fracture fixed with a dynamic hip screw. Non-union occurred with eventual breakage of the plate.

Management will depend on the timing of the cut-out and the pre-injury state of the patient. For those cases which occur within the early weeks after surgery, the most appropriate management is re-fixation. However, this can be a technically demanding procedure and should not be attempted by the inexperienced surgeon. The immediate postoperative and subsequent X-rays should be studied to determine how much of the femoral head bone remains. Generally re-insertion of the screw into an intact portion of the head is possible, fulfilling the criteria given earlier.

For those cases of cut-out which occur some weeks after the original surgery, it may be possible to leave the plate in place until the fracture is healed, then remove the implant. If extensive damage to the joint has occurred, a total hip replacement may subsequently be indicated.

Detachment of the plate from the femur

This is the second commonest technical problem encountered with the DHS, occurring in approximately 1–3% of patients. The diagnosis is easily confirmed on X-ray (Fig. 6.44).

This complication generally requires re-operation. The lag screw fixation of the proximal fragment can usually be left and a longer plate attached to the shaft. If the femoral shaft bone is markedly osteoporotic, augmentation of the screws, with cerclage wire or Partridge bands (plastic straps), may be helpful. Care

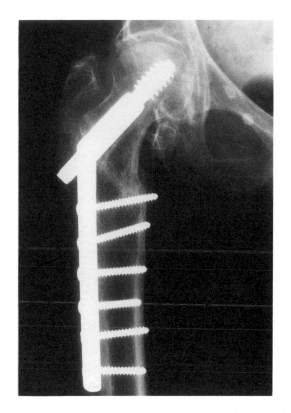

Fig. 6.46 A trochanteric fracture in which the dynamic hip screw ran out of slide (the DHS runs out of slide when the barrel comes to the end of the keyed or flattened section of the lag screw). The fracture line is still visible 1 year from injury.

must be taken to avoid the wires cutting through the bone, further comminuting the fracture. Reinforcement of the bone at the site of the screws with bone cement may also be used, although it will make any further re-operations technically difficult.

Non-union

Plate breakage, particularly if occurring some months after the fracture, will indicate that a non-union has developed. This is an infrequent complication of trochanteric fractures but more common in subtrochanteric fractures, where the incidence is approximately 2% (Fig. 6.45). It may also develop if the fracture ends are being held apart by a jammed

screw, unable to slide in the barrel of the plate (Fig. 6.46).

Non-union with or without implant failure is normally symptomatic, necessitating revision surgery. Surgical options include re-fixation with an extramedullary implant with bone grafting to the fracture site – a Medoff plate may be suitable for this. Alternatively, an intramedullary nail may be used which, if used without distal locking, gives a high stimulus to callus formation from weight-bearing.

Avascular necrosis

Avascular necrosis following an extracapsular fracture is rare. The blood supply to the proximal fragment is generally only compromised with basal fractures where the fracture line crosses the plane of capsular insertion. If

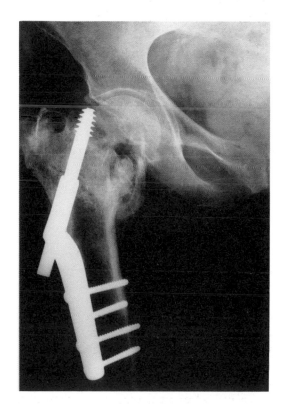

Fig. 6.47 A second fracture around the tip of a lag screw inserted for a trochanteric fracture.

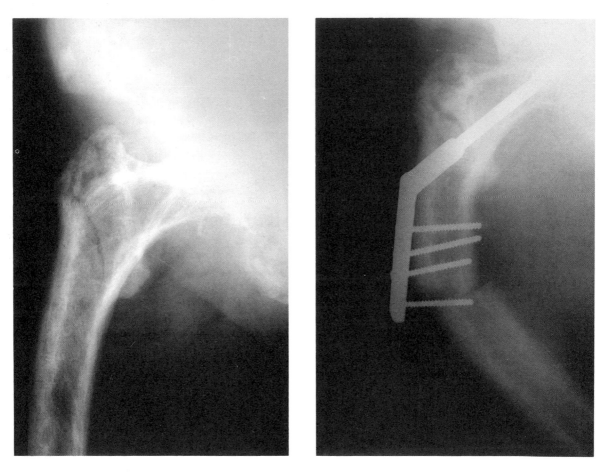

Fig. 6.48 A simple trochanteric fracture in a femur affected by Paget's disease treated with a dynamic hip screw. Further fracture occurred at the distal end of the plate.

significant collapse occurs and symptoms justify operation, arthroplasty will be necessary. This is a complex undertaking; the usual landmarks for insertion of the femoral component may be absent. A modular implant is often required to ensure correct limb length and soft-tissue tension.

Other complications

Fracture around the proximal end of the lag screw is rare, and generally caused by failure to insert the lag screw close enough to the joint, allowing a second fracture to occur (Fig. 6.47).

Fracture distal to the DHS plate is rare and generally only occurs in bone that is weakened by a pathological process such as tumour or Paget's disease (Fig. 6.48).

Implant removal

Routine removal of implants after hip fracture surgery is not normally indicated. Removal may be indicated after specific complications such as cut-out. For a patient who complains of persistent pain about the hip despite apparent successful and uncomplicated fracture healing, implant removal may be beneficial in improving symptoms in about 50% of cases.

Key references on fracture reduction

Clark DW, Ribbans WJ. Treatment of unstable intertrochanteric fractures of the femur: a prospective trial comparing anatomical reduction and valgus osteotomy. *Injury* 1990; 21:84–88.

Desjardins AL, Roy A, Paiement G *et al.* Unstable intertrochanteric fracture of the femur: a prospective randomised study comparing anatomical reduction and medial displacement osteotomy. *J Bone Joint Surg* 1993; 75–B:445–447.

Dimon JH, Hughston JC. Unstable intertrochanteric fractures of the hip. *J Bone Joint Surg* 1967; 49–A:440–450.

Hunter G, Krajbich I. Results of medial displacement osteotomy for unstable intertrochanteric fractures of the femur. *J Bone Joint Surg* 1979; 61–B:248.

Laros GS, Moore JF. Complications of fixation in intertrochanteric fractures. *Clin Orthop* 1974; 101:110–119.

Parker MJ. Valgus reduction of trochanteric fractures. *Injury* 1993; 24:313–316.

Sarmiento A, Williams EM. The unstable intertrochanteric fracture: treatment with a valgus osteotomy and I-beam nail-plate: a preliminary report of 100 cases. *J Bone Joint Surg* 1970; 52–A:1309–1318.

Key references on implant positioning

Davis TRC, Sher JL, Horsman A, Simpson M, Porter BB, Checketts RG. Intertrochanteric femoral fractures: mechanical failures after internal fixation. *J Bone Joint Surg* 1990; 72–B:26–31.

Kyle RF, Gustilo RB, Premer RF. Analysis of six hundred and twenty-two intertrochanteric hip fractures. *J Bone Joint Surg* 1979; 61–A:216–221.

Larsson S, Friberg S, Hansson L–I. Trochanteric fractures: influence of reduction and implant position on impaction and complications. *Clin Orthop* 1990; 259:130–139.

Mainds CC, Newman RJ. Implant failures in patients with proximal fractures of the femur treated with a sliding screw device. *Injury* 1989; 20:98–100.

Parker MJ. Cutting-out of the dynamic hip screw related to its position. *J Bone Joint Surg* 1992; 74–B:625.

Key references on specific fracture types

Cheng CL, Chow SP, Pun WK, Leong JCY. Long-term results and complications of cement augmentation in the treatment of unstable trochanteric fractures. *Injury* 1989; 20:134–138.

Hulleberg G, Finsen V. Removal of osteosynthesis material from healed hip fractures: indications and prognosis. *Ann Chir Gynecol* 1990; 79:161–164.

Kinast C, Bolhofner BR, Mast JW, Ganz R. Subtrochanteric fractures of the femur: results of treatment with the 95° condylar blade-plate. *Clin Orthop* 1989; 238:122–130.

Medoff RJ, Maes K. A new device for the fixation of unstable pertrochanteric fractures of the hip. *J Bone Joint Surg* 1991; 73–A:1992–1199.

Mullaji AB, Thomas TL. Low-energy subtrochanteric fractures in elderly patients: results of fixation with the sliding screw plate. *J Trauma* 1993; 34:56–61.

Parker MJ. Trochanteric hip fractures; fixation failure commoner with femoral medialisation, a comparison of 101 cases. *Acta Orthop Scand* 1996; 67:329–332.

Pogrund H, Kenan S, Franki U, Amir D. Another look at the pertrochanteric fracture of the femur: the relationship to osteoporosis. *Injury* 1987; 18:36–39.

7

Intramedullary fixation of extracapsular fractures

Indications

The recommended indications for intramedullary fixation of a hip fracture have been discussed in Chapter 2 and are listed below. As previously discussed, the routine use of an intramedullary implant for all trochanteric fractures is not recommended at present. This advice may change with the development and refinement of implants and surgical techniques.

Indications for intramedullary fixation

Low subtrochanteric fractures

Hip fracture with associated femoral shaft fracture

Pathological extracapsular fracture

Choice of implant

The more familiar type of femoral intramedullary nail consists of a nail inserted via the greater trochanter with one or more cross screws passed up through the femoral neck to the femoral head. A number of different types of nail are made; some of which are listed in Table 7.1.

There have been few comparative studies between these different implants, therefore it is not possible to be specific about which implant is the most appropriate.

Zickel nail

The use of this nail was first described by Zickel in 1976. It consists of a very solid angulated intramedullary nail with a stout side arm (Fig. 7.1). Conventionally it is inserted using an open procedure to expose the fracture. There is no facility for distal locking. Results of its use show that, once correctly inserted, fixation failure is exceptionally rare due to the high strength of the nail. Unfortunately, the nail can be technically demanding

---

Table 7.1 Different types of intramedullary implants that have been used for the fixation of extracapsular fractures

---

Gamma nail and long gamma nail
Grosse-Kempf interlocking nail
Kampala or Huckstep nail
Küntscher Y nail
Richards intramedullary hip screw
Russel-Taylor reconstruction nail
Vari-Wall reconstruction nail
Zickel nail

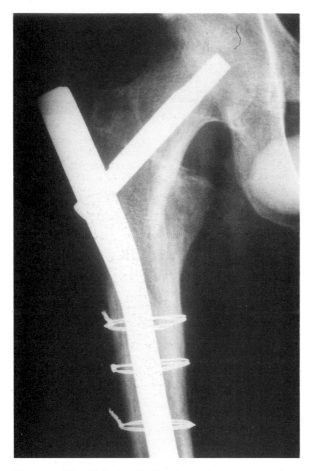

Fig. 7.1   The Zickel nail. Cerclage wires were used to assist in fracture reduction.

to use and removal of the nail may prove difficult, resulting in femoral fracture. Consequently this device is infrequently used now and cannot be recommended for the inexperienced trainee.

Küntscher Y nail

This consists of a straight Küntscher nail which is inserted through a neck nail. The insertion technique for this nail differs from other proximally inserted nails in that the neck nail is first inserted under X-ray control into the femoral head. An alignment jig is then attached to the neck nail to give the position for insertion of the straight Küntscher nail into the intramedullary cavity and through a

hole within the neck nail. There is no capacity for distal locking. The nail has shown similar results in comparison to the dynamic hip screw (DHS) in a randomized trial. However, overall failure rates were high in both groups in this study and there are few other published reports of the use of this type of nail.

Gamma nail

This is a more recently introduced implant. It is an angulated nail with a sliding cross screw (Fig. 7.2). It is designed to be inserted by a closed method and has facilities for distal locking to prevent rotation and shortening. The gamma nail has been extensively evaluated in a number of randomized trials, case series and mechanical studies. Results to date indicate that for trochanteric fracture the DHS appears to be the better implant; however, for subtrochanteric fractures the gamma nail is reported to have the advantages of reduced operating times and blood loss.

The original gamma nail is 200 mm long, the proximal diameter is 17 mm and there is a range of distal diameters of 11, 12 and 14 mm. The options of angles for the lag (cross) screw are 125°, 130° and 135°. The nail was initially made with a 10° bend just proximal to its midpoint but this was later changed to 8°. The long gamma nail has lengths of 340, 360, 380 and 400 mm, a distal diameter of 11 mm and proximal diameter of 17 mm (Fig. 7.3). Because it has to have a lateral curve to match the femur, there are left and right nails.

Ender's nails

Ender's nails are thin, flexible nails inserted through the medial femoral condyle and passed up the femoral medullary canal. Under X-ray control the nails are passed across the fracture into the proximal head/neck fragment, so the tips of the nails are in the subchondral bone. Usually three to five Ender's nails are inserted to fill up the medullary cavity. The postulated advantages are less bleeding during the operation and a reduced

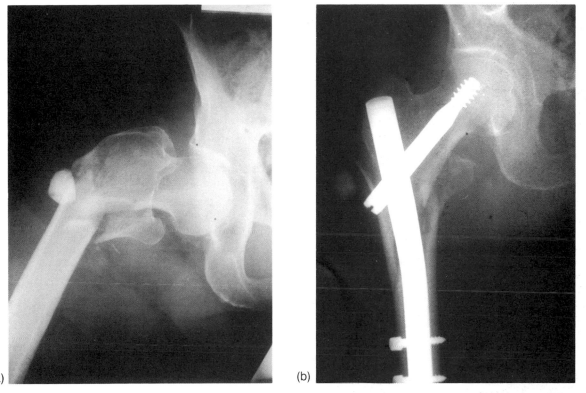

(a)   (b)

Fig. 7.2(a,b)   A three-part fracture at the level of the lesser trochanter treated with a gamma nail. The fracture has been fixed in a varus position (trabecular angle 145°), which has resulted in the lag screw being placed in an unacceptably high position. Some comminution of the fracture site occurred during nail insertion.

risk of infection. However, in comparative randomized studies with the screw plate, the Ender's nails have shown inferior results. The particular problems with Ender's nails were pain at the knee, backing out of the nails, loss of fracture position and a higher re-operation rate. Most centres have now abandoned Ender's nails and their use is not considered in this chapter.

Operative technique

The operative technique detailed here relates to intramedullary nails inserted by a closed technique via the greater trochanter, with insertion of a cross screw into the femoral neck and subsequent distal locking. The Zickel nail can be inserted by a closed technique, but this is technically difficult for an implant designed to be inserted with open exposure of the fracture. The Küntscher Y nail is unique in that the cross blade into the femoral neck has to be inserted first and its use is not described.

The insertion of an intramedullary nail is generally regarded as a more demanding technique than that for a screw plate, as described in Chapter 6. The intramedullary technique, however, can be mastered with practice and is an essential technique for fixation of long bone diaphyseal fractures.

Preoperative planning

Preoperative planning is an essential part of intramedullary fixation of an extracapsular fracture. In addition to an anteroposterior (AP) and lateral view of the fracture:

1 An X-ray of the pelvis is required, including the uninjured hip.

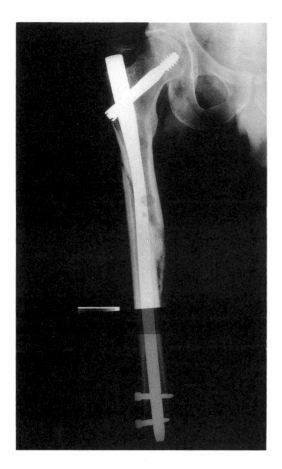

Fig. 7.3   A spiral subtrochanteric fracture of the femur fixed with a long gamma nail in good position.

1 Use a goniometer to predict the position of the lag screw within the femoral head. This will depend on the angle of implant used. Generally a 130° angle implant is preferable, as this reduces the risk of superior placement of the lag screw.
2 Determine if the site of lag screw insertion is above, at or below the fracture site.
3 Calculate the length of nail to be used. A nail of approximately 200 mm length is best avoided as it causes a stress point at the tip of the nail. As a rough guide there should be at least 100 mm of nail distal to the fracture or any femoral metastasis, to allow sound fixation of the distal locking screws. If in doubt, use a longer nail.
4 Calculate the diameter of the nail to be used. Generally it is recommended that a 12 mm nail is used.
5 Carefully check that there are no fissures in the proximal femoral shaft from the fracture extending distally; a longer nail may be indicated.
6 The degree of comminution of the fracture and position of the fragments are of less importance. When using a closed intramedullary nail technique, complete anatomical reduction of fragments is not as important as when using an extramedullary fixation.

Transparent templates from the implant manufacturers are helpful for correct preoperative planning. These templates have a 15% magnification to allow for the estimated degree of magnification that has occurred in taking the X-ray. The templates show the implant with 0° anteversion, thereby assuming that the X-ray has been taken in 10° of internal rotation; as this is rarely the case, the templates are inaccurate for determining the length of lag screw to be used.

2 For a pathological fracture an AP and lateral view of the entire length of the injured femur is required, to determine if any metastases are present down the femoral shaft.
3 If after plain X-rays there is still a suspicion of metastasis distal to the fracture site, a bone scan may be indicated.
4 If extensive metastasies are present throughout the femur, a full-length nail will be needed. An X-ray of uninjured femur incorporating a measuring scale is therefore required to enable the correct length of the nail to be determined.

Having obtained the appropriate X-rays the following elements should be studied:

Reduction of the fracture

One of the advantages with intramedullary fixation of extracapsular fractures is that it is normally possible to accomplish a closed reduction without exposure of the fracture

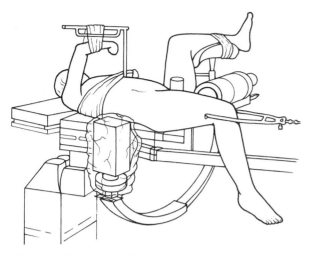

Fig. 7.4 Correct positioning of the patient and image intensifier to allow access to the area just proximal to the greater trochanter.

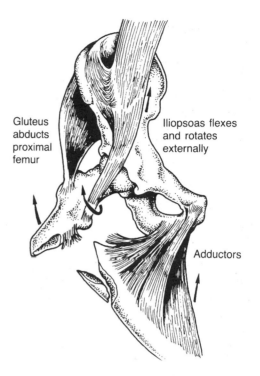

Fig. 7.5 For a subtrochanteric fracture the muscles attached to the trochanters pull the proximal fragment into flexion, abduction and external rotation.

site. This has the advantage of reducing the length of surgery, operative blood loss and the risk of sepsis. Furthermore, by not disturbing the fracture site and devascularizing bony fragments, the risk of non-union may be reduced.

The patient is positioned on a traction table as described in Chapter 4. For an intramedullary nailing procedure, particular care should be taken to ensure that there is access to the trochanteric area and above. The patient's trunk is curved towards the unaffected side. Ensure that the leg supports do not impede visualization of the entire length of the femur on both AP and lateral radiographs. For the lateral view of the femoral neck, a more transverse positioning of the image intensifier will allow better access to the superior-lateral part of the trochanteric and gluteal area (Fig. 7.4).

Fracture reduction should focus on restoring leg length, correcting any rotational deformity and angulation at the fracture site. Intermediate fragments may effectively be disregarded. On the fracture table traction is applied with the leg straight and the foot pointing upwards. After having alignment of the fracture in the AP view, it is often necessary to rotate the leg internally by 10–15°, to obtain full reduction of the fracture. The patella is therefore positioned either horizontally or with slightly internal rotation.

Unfortunately, particularly in subtrochanteric fractures, the pull of the flexor muscles can result in the proximal fragments being in a position of flexion, abduction and external rotation (Fig. 7.5). At the same time the femoral shaft is shortened and adducted. A number of measures may be used to overcome this:

1 Reposition the leg within the fracture table to align the bone ends.
2 Use external pressure to manipulate the fracture ends into alignment (Fig. 7.6).
3 Occasionally there is a tendency for the fracture to 'sink' posteriorly, and this can be visualized on the lateral image intensifier view (Fig. 7.7). This is more common in obese patients and those with trochanteric fractures. The angulation can be counteracted by an additional leg support such as a padded bar fixed to the leg

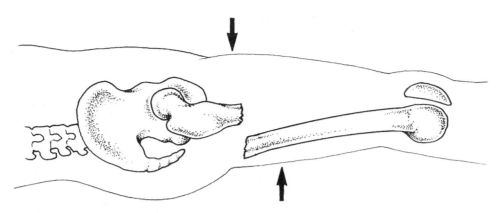

Fig. 7.6   External pressure may be used to reduce the fracture.

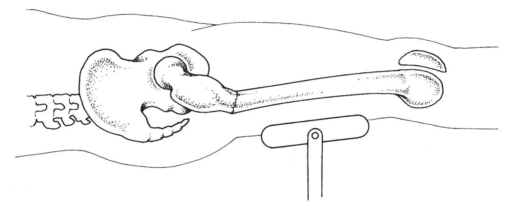

Fig. 7.7   Sag at the fracture site needs correction prior to nail insertion.

support bar. Alternatively an assistant can use a crutch or similar instrument to apply an anteriorly directed force to reduce the fracture.

4 Rarely, the problem is dorsal displacement of the distal fragment. A Steinmann pin may be inserted transversely across the femoral condyles to apply traction (Fig. 7.4). This enables traction to be released from the foot and the knee to be flexed, thereby reducing tension on the gastrocnemius muscle.

5 During the operation a short nail or a reduction rod is inserted into the proximal fragment to reduce the fracture (Fig. 7.8).

6 If all else fails, open reduction of the fracture is indicated. Sometimes this can

be done via a small incision at the level of the fracture site to enable a bone lever to be passed around the femur to manipulate the fracture. Failing this, a more extensive exposure of the fracture will be required,

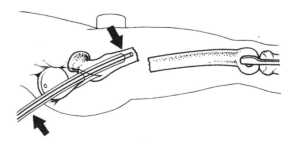

Fig. 7.8   A short intramedullary nail may be inserted into the proximal fragment during surgery to reduce the fracture.

using an approach as described for DHS fixation in Chapter 6. The fracture is held reduced by bone clamps applied each side of the fracture.

Incision

When performing the sterile cleaning and draping of the patient, it should be remembered that the position for the incision is more proximal than for application of a screw plate. However the site for the insertion of the distal locking screws must also be prepared.

If preferred, a Kirschner wire can be inserted percutaneously as a guide along and parallel to the front of the femoral neck (see Fig. 7.16). Its position is checked with the image intensifier. This guidewire can be used to orient where to make the incision and is later used to obtain the correct degree of rotation of the nail and position of the lag screw.

The incision is approximately 5–7 cm in length extending proximally from the greater trochanter (Fig. 7.9). Occasionally, particularly in the obese patient, the greater trochanter may be difficult to palpate. As a general guide, the greater trochanter is usually situated about 5 cm dorsal and 5 cm distal to the anterior superior iliac spine. Verification of the position using both the AP and lateral view with a marker held over the skin can be used.

The fascia lata is incised along the length of the incision. The fibres of gluteus medius arising from the greater trochanter are split for about 3–5 cm in the line of the muscle fibres, to expose the tip of the greater trochanter.

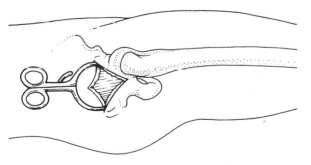

Fig. 7.9 Longitudinal incision extending for 5 cm proximal to the greater trochanter.

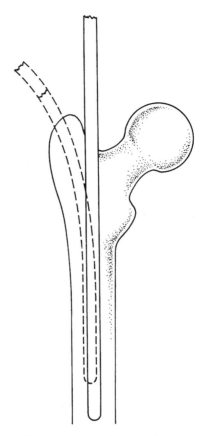

Fig. 7.10 Correct entry points on the anteroposterior radiograph for curved or straight intramedullary nails.

Entry point in the femur

The exact entry point into the greater trochanter will depend upon the type of nail to be used and the anatomy of the proximal femur. Considering first the hip as seen on the AP radiograph, the entry point will depend on whether the nail to be used is straight, angulated or curved when viewed from the front. For a straight nail such as the Küntscher or Huckstep nail, the entry hole is on the medial side of the greater trochanter, close to the base of the femoral neck in the piriformis fossa. For an angulated nail such as the gamma or Zickel, the entry hole is just lateral to the tip of the greater trochanter (Fig. 7.10).

On the lateral view the correct entry point will again depend on the type of nail used. When using a nail with a lateral curve such as the long gamma nail, Zickel, Russel-Taylor or

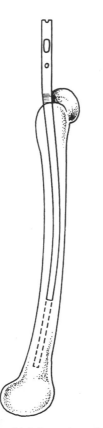

Fig. 7.11 For a nail which has a lateral curve the entry point becomes slightly posterior of centre.

Vari-Wall reconstruction nail, the nail will have to be made for left or right femur. For such nails the entry point becomes slightly posterior of centre (Fig. 7.11). For the 200 mm gamma nail which has an AP curve, but no lateral curve, the entry point is at the junction of the anterior third and posterior two-thirds on the greater trochanter. For completely straight nails that have no AP or lateral curves, such as the Küntscher or Huckstep nails, the anteversion of the femoral neck means that a central position in the piriformis fossa is chosen.

A summary of the entry points depending on the type of nail is shown in Figure 7.12. It is important to locate the correct entry site accurately. This may be by visualization if the fascia lata and abductor muscle are retracted, or by touch of the finger. Confirmation of the correct site on both the AP and lateral X-ray view is nevertheless recommended. The shape

of the greater trochanter and proximal femur is also variable and the entry point may need to be adjusted depending on the size and exact relationship of the greater trochanter to the medullary cavity.

The chosen entry point is made using a large curved awl through the greater trochanter into the medullary canal. The image intensifier is used to check that in the lateral plane the tip of the awl will reach the centre of the medullary canal.

An alternative method of entry into the medullary cavity is first to insert a guidewire through the correct entry point into the medullary cavity. AP and lateral X-rays are taken to check that it is in the correct position. A cannulated reamer similar to that used for DHS fixation is then passed over the guidewire to ream the proximal 4–5 cm or femur.

Insertion of the guidewire

Next a reamer guidewire with a ball tip is passed distally from the trochanteric region, across the fracture into the shaft of the femur (Fig. 7.13). A ball-tipped guidewire is used in case one of the reamers breaks; it can be removed by pulling on the guidewire. The guidewire is best inserted by hand with the aid of a Jacobs chuck. The surgeon should be able to tell that the guidewire is within the femur from the correct amount of resistance as it is pushed distally.

Difficulties may be encountered in getting the tip of the guidewire across the fracture site. The following points may help:

1 An unscrubbed assistant can apply external pressure to the leg to reduce the fracture, whilst the guidewire is passed across the fracture site.
2 Bend the tip of the guidewire by 5–10° at 2 cm from the tip, so that it can be aimed in the correct direction across the fracture site.
3 Insert a narrow-diameter nail or reduction rod into the proximal part of the fracture. Use this to reduce the fracture, allowing the guidewire to be pushed across the fracture (Fig. 7.8).

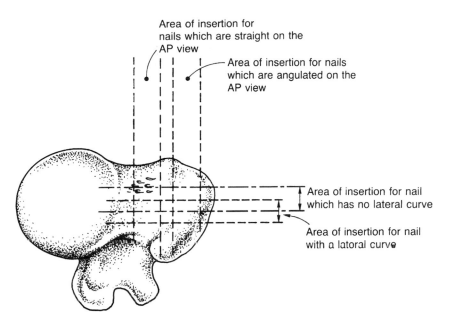

Area of insertion for
nails which are straight on the
AP view

Area of insertion for nails
which are angulated on the
AP view

Area of insertion for nail
which has no lateral curve

Area of insertion for nail
with a lateral curve

Fig. 7.12   Superior view of femur to show the different insertion points depending on the type of nail to be used.

4 If all else fails, the fracture site has to be exposed and the fracture reduced openly, as described above.

Reaming of the femur

With flexible power reamers the shaft of the femur is reamed. The following points should be remembered:

1 Flexible reamers should never be used in reverse, as this causes the reamers to unwind and become jammed in the femoral canal.
2 Start reaming with a 9 mm diameter and then increase in 0.5 mm increments. In patients with a wide medullary canal, however, reaming can often start with an 11 or 12 mm diameter. Over-reaming the femur from the diameter of the nail to be used by a 1–1.5 mm minimum is mandatory. For the gamma nail over-reaming by 2 mm is recommended. In wide osteoporotic femur reaming of the shaft may not be required.
3 For the gamma nail where there is expansion of the proximal part of the nail to accommodate the lag screw, the trochanteric region down to the level of the lesser trochanter should be reamed to 17 mm. This reaming is essential to reduce the risk of operative femoral fracture.
4 Whilst reaming, ensure that the guidewire is not displaced laterally, as this may result in an asymmetrically placed nail.
5 For the majority of cases a 12 mm diameter nail is sufficient irrespective of femoral width, therefore reaming is to 13.5 or 14 mm. With modern implants such as the gamma nail, a 12 mm diameter is strong enough to withstand loading, whilst the risk of intraoperative fracture is reduced.
6 Further reaming from the point where the reamer starts to bite on the cortical bone is not recommended (Fig. 7.14). In elderly osteoporotic patients there is usually cortical bone re-absorption which has widened the medullary canal and reaming of cortical bone can weaken the femur.

Insertion of the nail

The selected nail (at least 1.5 mm smaller than the reamed diameter) is assembled with its specially designed introducer jig. The surgeon should be aware of how the alignment jig of the particular nail that is being used fits together.

Depending on the type of nail, the ball-tipped guidewire may need to be changed to a straight wire. A plastic exchange sheath may be used to accomplish this without losing the position of the guidewire within the femur. For nails which are cannulated to a sufficient diameter to allow the ball-tipped guidewire to pass through the nail, this is not necessary.

The nail is then passed over the guidewire into the femur. When inserting the nail it is important not to use excessive force. This has been found to be particularly important for the gamma nail, which must be inserted by hand and never hammered into place. Insertion is usually facilitated by anterior–posterior

rotating movements while pushing the nail downwards.

The nail is introduced until the lag screw holes are lined up with the direction of the centre of the femoral neck. On the AP view they are visible as crescent shapes on the contour of the nail (Fig. 7.15).

If a percutaneous wire has been positioned along the femoral neck, the shaft of the nail introducer should be parallel to this guidewire (Fig. 7.16). This guarantees the correct degree of rotation to allow the lag screw to be positioned with the correct angle of anteversion into the femoral neck.

If it is not possible to push the nail into the femoral canal with ease, then the nail must be withdrawn and either further reaming undertaken or a thinner nail used. Forceful hammering of the nail must be avoided, otherwise fracture of the femoral shaft can occur.

After positioning the intramedullary nail, the reaming guidewire is removed using a Jacobs chuck. Next the targeting device corresponding to the nail is assembled on to the side of the introducer. In order to reduce any slackness within the targeting device it is important that the connecting bolts are fully tightened. Frequently the weight of this targeting device is such that it has to be supported by hand, otherwise the nail may slowly rotate externally as the device sinks down.

Positioning of the femoral lag screw (or cross screws)

The nail's position determines the tract of the threaded guidewire for the lag screw. The

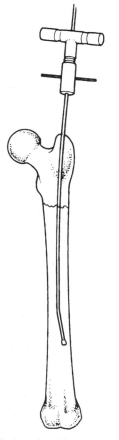

Fig. 7.13 A ball-tipped guidewire is passed across the fracture site.

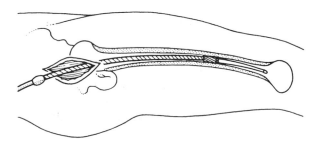

Fig. 7.14 In an osteoporotic femur the cortical bone must not be reamed. Reaming to a diameter to allow a 12 mm nail to be used is usually sufficient.

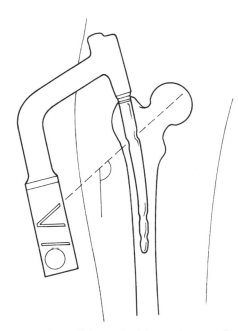

Fig. 7.15 The nail is pushed into place until the lag screw holes indicate that the lag screw will be inserted into the centre of the femoral head. This is best measured on the image intensifier screen.

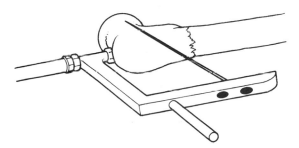

Fig. 7.16 A guidewire placed parallel to and superior to the femoral neck should be parallel to the transverse bar of the introducer.

depth to which the nail has been inserted determines the position of the lag screw on the AP radiograph. If it appears, from the position of the lag screw hole as seen on the AP radiograph, that the screw will be superiorly placed, the nail must be pushed further into the femur. This may involve removing the nail to allow further reaming of the femur. Changing the nail to one with a smaller angle for the lag screw does little to lower the screw tip within the femoral head.

On the lateral radiograph the lag screw must be inserted into the centre of the femoral head. The position of the lag screw is altered by rotating the nail within the femur. As mentioned earlier, a guidewire inserted percutaneous along the femoral neck may be used to assist in determining the correct degree of rotation (Fig. 7.16).

The skin at the site of lag screw insertion on the lateral side of the thigh is incised. With the aid of the target jig, the soft-tissue protector and lag screw guide sleeve are passed through the incision down to the femur. With the teeth of the guide sleeve firmly engaging the femur, the lateral femoral cortex is perforated with an awl. Using an obturator within the soft-tissue protector a guidewire mounted on a Jacobs chuck is inserted.

The position of the guidewire should be checked in both the AP and the lateral planes. The tip of the guidewire should be just below the centre of the femoral head on the AP view and central on the lateral view (Fig. 7.17) to minimize the risk of the lag screw cutting out. If the guidewire is too superior it must be removed and the nail pushed further down the femur. If the guidewire is too anterior or posterior it must be reinserted after the rotation of the nail has been corrected.

Once the correct position of the guidewire has been achieved, the length of lag screw required is obtained using a measuring gauge. For the gamma nail the measurement from the gauge is the same as that for the lag screw, as the threaded portion of the guidewire is not included in the measurement. For other types of implant, however, a subtraction of 5–10 mm may be needed to allow the tip of the lag screw to be 5–10 mm for the joint line. The track for the lag screw is drilled using a reamer with an adjustable stop. The depth of drilling should however be confirmed by the image intensifier. In most instances the path for the lag screw can be reamed by hand using a Jacobs chuck, which is generally easy in osteoporotic patients (Fig. 7.18). If a power drill is used, care is needed not to drill into the hip joint itself.

The lag screw is then inserted to a depth such that its tip is about 5 mm from the joint

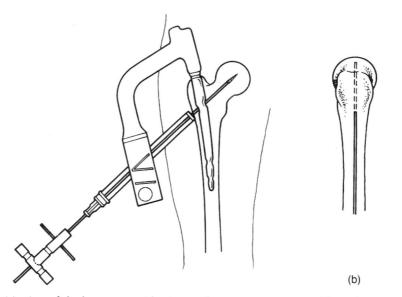

(b)

Fig. 7.17   Correct positioning of the lag screw guidewire on the anteroposterior and lateral views. Malpositioning of the guidewire must not be accepted as this increases the risk of lag screw cut-out.

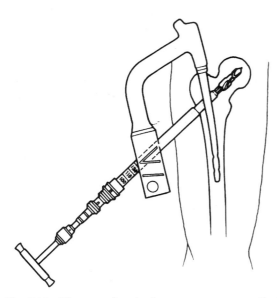

Fig. 7.18   The tract for the lag screw can normally be reamed by hand. Note that for the gamma nail the correct setting of the reamer is made by reading from the side nearest the drill tip (100 mm in this case). This is the opposite to that for a dynamic hip screw.

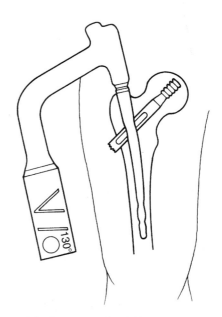

Fig. 7.19   The lag screw should be 5 mm from the joint line and protrude slightly from the lateral femoral cortex.

line. For the gamma nail a lag screw 5 mm longer than that reading from the measuring gauge should be used. This allows the lateral end of the lag screw to protrude slightly from the lateral femoral cortex to retain rotational stability (Fig. 7.19). If a Russel-Taylor or Vari-

Wall reconstruction nail is being used, then two cross screws are used instead of a single lag screw (Fig. 7.20).

Depending on the type of nail used, a set screw may need to be inserted into the top of the nail to engage a groove along the shaft of the lag screw. This prevents rotation of the lag screw. With the gamma nail the lag screw insertion handle should be placed parallel to the shaft of the femur. This enables a locking set screw to be inserted into the proximal end of the nail. This is tightened and then unscrewed one-quarter of a turn to ensure free sliding of the lag screw.

Technical problems which may be encountered at this time are:

1 If a power drill is used to insert the guidewire without perforating the lateral femoral cortex, it may bend and end up too high in the femoral head. Subsequent reaming with the step drill over this guidewire will result in jamming of the reamer.

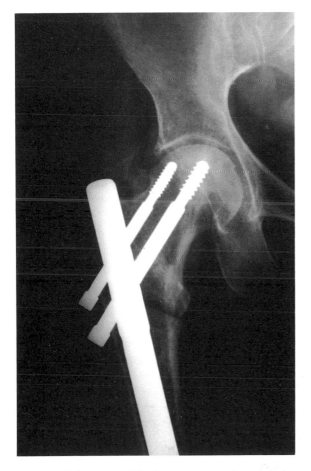

Fig. 7.20 The Russel-Taylor reconstruction nail has two cross-screws. In this case the nail should have been pushed a little more distally into the femur so that the lower screw is resting on the calcar and the upper screw is not placed so superiorly.

This problem is avoided if the lateral femoral cortex is perforated with an awl or drilled before the guidewire is inserted.

2 When the step drill is used to make the track for the lag screw, the nail and guidewire may be pushed proximally. This should be counteracted by pushing distally on the nail introducer during drilling.

3 In some cases repositioning of the guidewire may be difficult due to its tendency to follow its old false track. The guidewire may be removed and the step drill used freehand through the targeting device. In these cases it is important to avoid rotation of the target device to achieve the correct anteversion for the lag screw and to screen repeatedly in both the AP and lateral radiographs whilst drilling.

4 In some comminuted fractures there is difficulty in passing the guidewire into the centre of the femoral head, because the fracture is displayed posteriorly by gravity on the suspended leg. This can be counteracted by lifting the whole system through the nail insertion jig. Alternatively, the whole trochanter area can be lifted by the hand of an assistant or maybe through a femoral support, as described previously. This will keep the femoral shaft, neck and head in a straight line, enabling the guidewire to be passed to the centre of the head.

5 In the lateral view the targeting device can sometimes hamper the positioning of the guidewire by obscuring the view of the femoral head on the image intensifier. To overcome this the image intensifier can be rotated by a few degrees upwards or downwards to an oblique position, to give a full view of the guidewire. If necessary, the correct position of the guidewire can be extrapolated from the different images. It is also possible gently to use the targeting device as a handle and make small anterior and posterior rotations, to see how the targeting device projects along the mid axes of the femoral neck and up into the centre of the femoral head. This problem has lately been overcome by

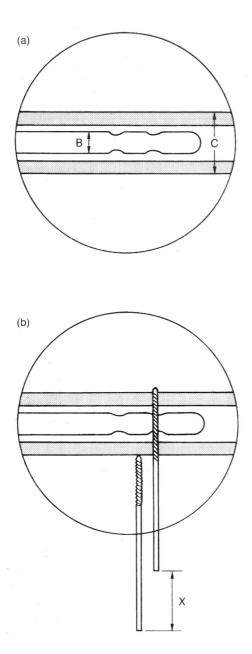

Fig. 7.21 Alternative methods of measuring the length of distal locking screws utilizing the image intensifier in the anteroposterior (AP) position. (a) Measurements are taken from the X-ray screen of an AP view of the nail at the side of the distal locking holes. The known diameter of the nail (A) is used to correct for any magnification. The diameter of the nail (B) and the width of the femur (C) on the X-ray screen are measured. The length of screw to be used is A/B×C. (b) The drill tip is positioned so that it just protrudes from the medial femoral cortex on the AP view. A drill of the same length is used to determine the length of drill within the femur (×).

using radiopaque materials for the targeting device.

Distal locking of the nail

The potential advantages of distal locking are:

1 To reduce pain on walking. Clinical experience suggests that, even for stable trochanteric fractures, distal locking reduces groin and thigh pain.
2 To provide additional rotational stability, which is particularly relevant in subtrochanteric fractures. For trochanteric fractures the lateral protrusion of the lag screw in the distal fragment should provide some rotational stability.
3 To control the leg length with a comminuted subtrochanteric fracture. This is particularly useful if there is a disparity between the diameter of the nail and the femur.
4 If distal locking is not performed and the lag screw is short such that it does not protrude from the lateral femoral cortex. Then with weight-bearing the whole assembled nail, together with a proximal part of the fracture, can be pushed distally into the femoral shaft. This may result in the lateral femoral cortex preventing the lag screw from sliding. Further collapse around the fracture site may result in cutting out of the lag screw.

The arguments against distal locking are:

1 Mechanical studies indicate that distal locking is superfluous for stable two- and three-part trochanteric fractures.
2 Rotational stability can be tested by trying to rotate the nail after the lag screw has been inserted. If there is good resistance against rotational forces distal locking may be unnecessary.
3 Without any distal locking there is a kind of dynamization of the whole system during weight-bearing.

On balance therefore, distal locking with

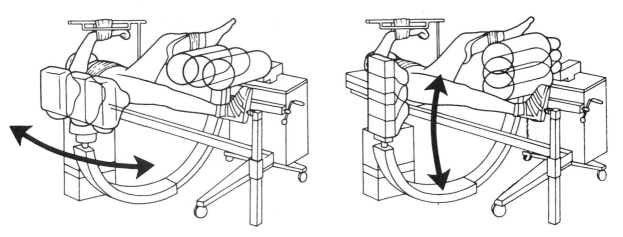

Fig. 7.22 The image intensifier is placed at 90° to the nail and the rotation of the leg or the angulation of the image intensifier adjusted to obtain a view of the distal locking screw holes as a perfect circle.

two screws is generally recommended, especially if the fracture is subtrochanteric.

Distal locking of short nails

For short nails such as the 200 mm gamma nail, the same targeting device used for insertion of the lag screw is utilized to insert the distal locking screws. The skin incision and all preparations for the screw holes are made through the targeting device.

The following points are important:

1 There must be no looseness between the jig components or at its connection to the nail. Any laxity within the jig can cause the locking screws to miss the nail holes.
2 A sharp pointed awl should be used to indent the femoral cortex for a few millimetres before drilling. If the drill is used first it may slide posteriorly off the rounded outer cortex of the femur. In more osteoporotic patients it is possible to push the awl all the way through both cortices by hand. However, do not use excessive force with the awl as it may result in crack fracture.

After drilling, measurement of the distal screw length is made with a depth gauge. If this is not available, alternative methods of determining the correct screw length are shown in Figure 7.21.

Distal locking of long nails

Whilst there are a number of devices available to assist distal screw insertion, the majority of surgeons have not found these helpful and adopt the so-called freehand technique.

First the image intensifier is placed in the lateral view at right angles to the longitudinal axis of the femoral shaft. The rotation of the leg is adjusted until the holes for the distal locking screws in the nail appear as perfect circles (Fig. 7.22). If they are oval, either the image intensifier or the rotation of the leg must be adjusted until a complete circle is obtained.

A thin sharp pointed awl is then introduced from the side and positioned on the lateral side of the leg with its point in the middle of the round hole on the image intensifier view. Next a stab incision is made down to the bone. The awl is repositioned so its tip lies on the bone with its point positioned in the centre of the round hole on the image intensifier (Fig. 7.23). Without moving the position of the tip of the awl, it is brought into a 90° position perpendicular to the long axis of the femur. By twisting movements the awl is used to perforate the femoral cortex and can often be felt to go into the distal locking hole of the nail. The awl is removed and a drill passed through the hole made to drill the opposite cortex, using the image intensifier in the AP view to confirm correct positioning.

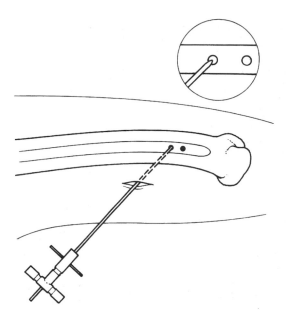

Fig. 7.23 Freehand distal locking to locate the correct site for screw insertion. The tip of the awl must be maintained in the centre of image of the distal locking hole, which is seen as a perfect circle.

The disadvantage with the freehand technique is the close proximity of the surgeon's hands to the radiation exposure of the image intensifier. To reduce this, radiopaque aiming devices have been developed, such as the radiolucent drill. This is held by its handle whilst the drill tip is positioned within the centre of the perfect circle of the distal locking screw hole. Two circles of the drill head are then aligned with the perfect circle, indicating that the drill is in line with the distal locking holes (Fig. 7.24). An alternative targeting device uses a laser beam fitted to the C arm of the image intensifier to produce a red light on the leg, which is seen as a cross on the X-ray screen. Once the image intensifier is correctly positioned the incision and perforation of the lateral femoral cortex are performed under guidance of the red laser beam.

After the drill hole for the distal locking screw has been made, the correct screw length may be determined by using the measuring gauge or alternatively the method shown in Figure 7.21. A screw of appropriate length is then inserted, with tapping of the threads if necessary.

Closure of the wound

Generally it is only necessary to suture the skin incisions, although occasionally a few interrupted sutures may be used to close the fascia lata. The value of using a vacuum drain to the proximal wound is debatable. Conventionally one drain is recommended to reduce the risk of haematoma formation; however, some surgeons feel that a vacuum drain may cause excessive bleeding from the area of femoral reaming.

Postoperative management

The rehabilitation and postoperative management after gamma nail osteosynthesis are similar to that for DHS fixation (Chapter 6). For the majority of fractures, weight-bearing should be allowed with encouragement of

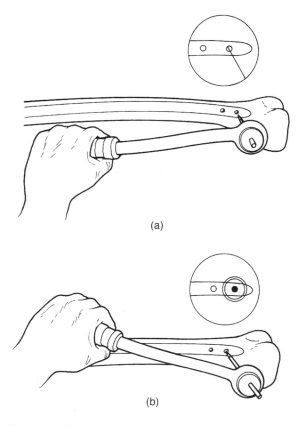

(a)

(b)

Fig. 7.24 Distal locking using a radiolucent targeting drill.

early mobilization. No restriction on hip movement is necessary. If used, a drain should not be retained for more than 48 h.

Complication of intramedullary fixation

Operative fracture around the nail

Intraoperative fracture of the femur has been reported to occur in approximately 3% of gamma nail fixations (Fig. 7.2). Inadequate reaming of the femur is normally the cause, in conjunction with excessive force when inserting the nail. An alternative cause may be because the lateral cortical bone around the lag screw is not load-protected by a barrel, as with the DHS a fissure in this area may more readily extend. With attention to surgical detail intraoperative comminution or extension of the fracture should be rare.

Treatment may be by stabilizing the fracture with the distal locking screws. If a short nail was the intended implant, it may be necessary to use a longer implant to obtain a more secure fixation distal to the fracture.

Later fracture around the nail

This typically occurs at the tip of the nail and has been reported to occur in approximately 2% of fixations using a short nail. The cause is thought to be due to the load-bearing capacity of the device which results in a stress point just below the tip of the nail. Alternative causes may be asymmetrical reaming of the mid-shaft of the femur contributing to cortical weakening or the high inherent stiffness of some implants, imparting a non-physiological strain on the proximal femur.

Treatment of this complication is demanding. Conservative treatment with traction may be used but most authors have favoured revision surgery using a longer intramedullary nail.

Rarely, fracture can occur proximal to the implant. Nails which are locked with an oblique cross screw passed distally and

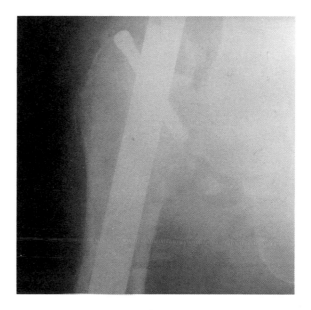

Fig. 7.25 Fracture around the proximal locking screw of an intramedullary nail used to treat a subtrochanteric fracture.

medially between the trochanters are inadequate for subtrochanteric fracture, as there is a risk of the fracture extending around the proximal locking screw (Fig. 7.25). The rigidity of the nail may also result in an intracapsular fracture (Fig. 7.26).

Cut-out of the implant

Studies to date have found that the incidence of cut-out for intramedullary fixation is comparable to that for DHS fixation, with an overall incidence of 3%. Treatment is as discussed in Chapter 6.

Non-union of the fracture

The incidence of non-union of subtrochanteric fractures after intramedullary fixation is approximately 3%. Without treatment the nail will eventually break, making revision surgery difficult.

Treatment may initially be by removing the distal locking screws to 'dynamize' the fracture, with encouragement of weight-bearing.

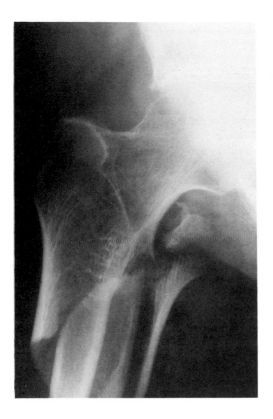

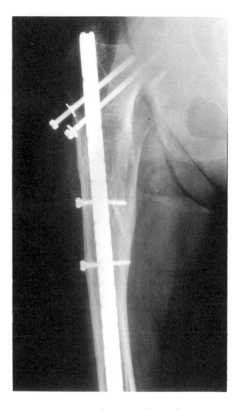

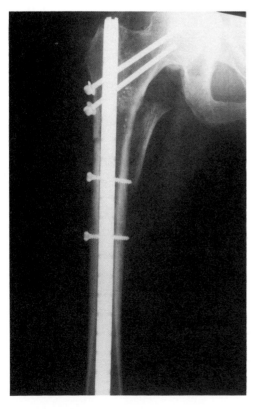

Fig. 7.26   A Huckstep nail used to treat a subtrochanteric fracture. The patient later developed a subcapital fracture around the thin proximal locking screws.

If this fails, revision of fixation, possibly using another intramedullary nail or with bone grafting at the fracture site, is indicated.

Key references

Calvert PT. The gamma nail: a significant advance of a passing fashion? *J Bone Joint Surg* 1992; **74–B**:329–331.

Davis TRC, Sher JL, Checketts RG, Porter BB. Intertrochanteric fractures of the femur: a prospective study comparing the use of the Küntscher-Y nail and a sliding hip screw. *Injury* 1988; **19**:421–426.

Fornander P, Thorngren K-G, Törnqvist H, Ahrengart L, Lingren U. Swedish experience with the Gamma nail versus sliding hip screw in 209 randomised cases. *Int J Orthop Trauma* 1994; **4**: 118–122.

Grosse A, Favreul E, Taglang G. The long gamma nail experience: 79 cases. *Orthopaedics* 1994; **2**:3.

Parker MJ, Robinson CM. Gamma nail versus

sliding hip screw for the treatment of extracapsular fracture of the proximal femur. In: Gillespie WJ, Madhok R, Swiontkowski M, Robinson CM, Murray GD (eds) Musculoskeletal injuries Module of The Cochrane Database of Systematic Reviews. Available in The Cochrane Library [database on disk and CDROM]. The Cochrane Collaboration; Oxford: Update software: 1996. BMJ publishing group, London.

Schatzker J, Waddell JP. Subtrochanteric fractures of the femur. *Orthop Clin North Am* 1980; **11**:539–554.

Zickel RE. An intramedullary fixation device for the proximal part of the femur. *J Bone Joint Surg* 1976; **58–A**:866–872.

8

Arthroplasty

The question of whether to treat as intracapsular hip fracture by internal fixation or arthroplasty is discussed in Chapter 2. Once the choice has been made to replace rather than reduce and fix the femoral head, the next decisions are:

1 The type of prosthesis to be used.
2 Whether the prosthesis should be cemented in place.
3 The surgical approach.

This chapter describes the most commonly used prostheses and surgical approaches. It must be emphasized that there is no one correct approach or prosthesis. Far more important is the technical accuracy of the surgery. Moreover, it is important not to fall into the trap of comparing hip fracture patients with those undergoing total arthroplasty for osteoarthritis. The two groups are very different and what may be best for one is not necessarily appropriate for the other.

Choice of prosthesis

When considering the prosthesis the choice is between a solid head prosthesis, bipolar hemiarthroplasty or a primary total hip arthroplasty.

Solid head prosthesis

The most commonly used prostheses in the UK today are still the Moore and Thompson designs, developed over 40 years ago (Fig. 8.1). Both have a solid head and differ in the shape of the stem and angle of the collar. Both were introduced before the advent of bone cement, although nowadays the Thompson stem is frequently cemented in place. The Moore stem – hardly a sophisticated uncemented design by modern standards – does have reasonable rotational stability and is normally used without cement. Despite being invented in the 1940s it still remains one of the most commonly used hemiarthroplasty in the

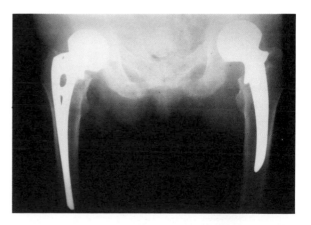

Fig. 8.1 A Moore (left) and Thompson (right) prosthesis used here without cement.

UK. The uncemented Thompson stem has less stability within the femoral shaft and should never be used without cement with a posterior approach, because of a tendency to dislocation.

Bipolar prosthesis

The bipolar head design (Fig. 8.2), of an inner bearing designed to allow movement within the head assembly, rather than between prosthesis and acetabulum, is still of unproven value. Intended to reduce the incidence of acetabular erosion, the most recent comparisons in those aged over 80 years, failed to find any benefit for the bipolar. For those aged less than 80 years, there may be a small reduction in the incidence of acetabular erosion, but further clinical studies are required to confirm this.

This type of prosthesis is more expensive and adds to the complexity of the operation. If dislocation subsequently occurs, there is an increased risk that open reduction will be necessary. The authors feel that, for the 'younger' patients in whom a bipolar prosthesis may possibly be advantageous to a unipolar hemiarthroplasty, reduction and internal fixation should be the initial treatment of choice. The value of a bipolar hemiarthroplasty is therefore questionable; furthermore it is not an implant to be used by the inexperienced surgeon.

Total hip replacement

This has very limited indications in the primary management of hip fracture. Moreover, it should not be undertaken by junior surgeons unfamiliar with the complexities of this procedure. Correct cement technique, accurate alignment of the acetabular component and proper soft-tissue dissection and closure are essential to ensure a reasonable chance of lasting success.

The possibility of damage to the acetabulum, as with a pathological fracture, Paget's

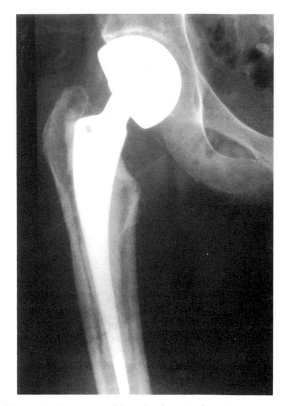

Fig. 8.2   A cemented bipolar hemiarthroplasty.

disease or coexisting arthritis with a hip fracture, may however justify total hip arthroplasty. In the younger patient with a displaced intracapsular fracture, if fracture reduction cannot be achieved by closed means, open reduction and bone grafting or fixation in the best possible position is generally preferable to total hip arthroplasty.

To date studies of the use of total hip replacement in hip fracture patients have demonstrated markedly inferior results to that following replacement of arthritic hip (hip arthrosis). The early complication rate is higher, especially dislocation, with an incidence of around 10%. Long-term implant survival rates are also inferior for total hip replacement in hip fracture patients, in comparison to arthritic patients.

Use of cement

Since Sir John Charnley's original work, there has been little doubt that polymethylmethacrylate bone cement improves bonding and hence stability between the prosthetic stem and femoral shaft. Clinical studies have shown that this results in less residual pain in the hip, increased mobility and a reduced revision rate from loosening of the femoral stem. Moreover the enthusiasm for uncemented total joint replacement has diminished since the simplistic concept of cement disease as the main cause of aseptic loosening has been replaced by particle disease. So can there be any justification for the use of an uncemented hemiarthroplasty? The answer is yes, for a number of reasons, not least because of the differences between hip fracture patients and the osteoarthritic patient undergoing total hip replacement.

The fracture patient is older, more frail, undergoing an emergency procedure and usually suffering from coexisting medical problems. Even with modern anaesthetic techniques, the insertion of cement is associated with a risk of hypotensive collapse and cardiac arrest. The extent of this risk is related to the physical state of the patient: for a relatively fit patient with no cardiovascular or respiratory disease with normal electrolytes the risk is minimal. However, for a frail elderly patient with evidence of cardiac or respiratory disease, the risk of major complications with cement rises to 2–4%. The osteoporotic femur is also less suited to effective cement techniques; pressurization can be difficult in a wide femur and may bypass or force the cement restrictor distally. The presence of cement will complicate any revision procedure and cemented arthroplasty in hip fracture patients has a much higher rate of loosening in comparison to arthroplasty for hip arthritis.

The converse is also true, in so far as the osteoporotic femur is unlikely to provide the initial primary stability necessary for an uncemented stem to gain osseous integration. Newer designs of stem such as the Bateman come in a variety of sizes, with the aim of achieving a better interference fit between stem and shaft. Unfortunately, the weaker, more brittle bone in these patients leads to a higher incidence of fractures with a tighter-fitting prosthesis. This therefore leads many surgeons to continue with the traditional uncemented Moore prosthesis.

In conclusion, while cemented hemiarthroplasty makes for a more stable fixation, it is a greater risk of complications and any subsequent surgery will be more difficult.

Advantages of cement	Disadvantages of cement
Less residual pain	More demanding operation
Increased mobility	Increased mortality
Reduced revision rate	Makes revision surgery harder

Surgical approaches to the hip joint

Specific factors that must be borne in mind when deciding on the surgical approach for hip fracture surgery are:

1 Early mobilization is essential.
2 Postoperative restrictions should be kept to the absolute minimum. Ideally there should be none.
3 Postoperative dislocation must be avoided as far as possible by accurate surgery rather than ill-conceived restrictions, such as periods of bed rest postoperatively.

These factors mean in practical terms that tissue dissection must be kept to a minimum by using a surgical approach between muscle groups or splitting rather than dividing muscle fibres. Bony dissection, removing sections of greater trochanter, should be avoided. Capsulotomy rather than capsulectomy is the rule, to limit instability.

The hip joint can be approached surgically from any direction – anterior, anterolateral, lateral, posterolateral, posterior and even medially (Fig. 8.3). However the trainee surgeon need only be familiar with one or two approaches. Any approach will be a compromise between the necessary exposure and excessive surgical dissection. In hip fracture surgery, the most appropriate exposures are

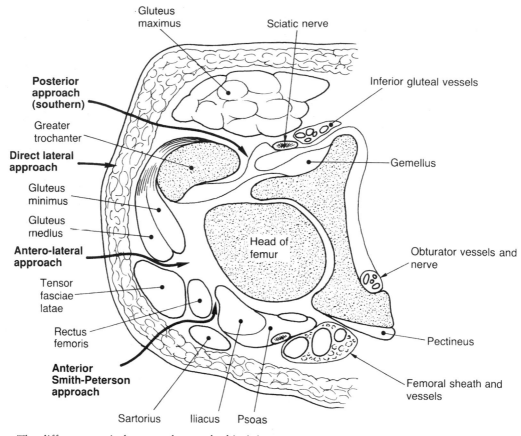

Fig. 8.3   The different surgical approaches to the hip joint.

the various lateral approaches or the posterior approach. None has been shown conclusively to be superior as there are advantages and disadvantages to both. Furthermore the type of prosthesis to be used must be taken into consideration.

Approaches to the hip

With the anterior approach described by Smith-Petersen in 1949, the hip is approached in the plane between sartorius and tensor fasciae latae, then between iliopsoas and rectus femoris. Other than for biopsy of the hip, this approach is rarely used and is not appropriate for arthroplasty.

The anterolateral approach to the hip involves developing the plane between tensor

fascia lata anteriorly and gluteus medius posteriorly, down on to the anterior capsule.

A variety of lateral approaches to the hip joint have been described. These differ mainly in the proportions of gluteus medius and vastus lateralis that are detached. The first, coinciding with the introduction of hip arthroplasty, was the McFarland and Osborne approach described in 1954. This procedure involves peeling the gluteus medius muscle forwards off the greater trochanter in continuity with a portion of vastus lateralis attached to the inferior border of the greater trochanter and linea aspera. The whole muscle mass is displaced forwards like elevating a bucket handle. The underlying gluteus minimus tendon is divided to expose the hip joint.

The Hardinge approach published in 1982 entails detaching the bulk of gluteus medius, but only a small portion of the vastus lateralis, from the greater trochanter. The posterior tendinous portion of gluteus medius is left attached to the greater trochanter and provides an anchoring point when reattaching the muscle after the procedure.

Several other lateral approaches to the hip have been described. The Stracathro approach is a modification of the McFarland-Osborne technique – instead of the conjoined tendon of gluteus medius and vastus lateral being reflected forwards from the greater trochanter, both muscles are split vertically in line of their fibres. Two slices of trochanter are elevated, one anteriorly and one posteriorly. The muscle attached to these slices is then retracted to expose the gluteus minimus. This muscle is detached to expose the hip capsule. Such an approach in osteoporotic bone of a hip fracture patient runs the risk of damaging the proximal femur. This technique is not recommended unless the surgeon is thoroughly experienced in the approach.

A further modification of the McFarland-Osborne approach was described by Dall in 1986. The proximal two-thirds of gluteus medius and the vastus lateralis are reflected forwards with a slice of anterior portion of trochanter. The reflection of the whole of the vastus lateralis from its posterior insertion, rather than longitudinal splitting of the muscle belly, avoids denervating the posterior half and reduces bleeding from vessels within the muscle. The reflection of an anterior slice of the trochanter is a disadvantage and it must be carefully reattached to avoid later separation. A more recent modification of the lateral approach by Frndak and colleagues (1993) involved splitting gluteus medius more anteriorly.

The classic Charnley approach involves detaching the greater trochanter with the gluteus medius muscle. This gives an excellent exposure; however, such a wide exposure is not necessary for hip fracture surgery. Surgery will be excessively prolonged by reattaching the greater trochanter and there are frequently problems with healing of the detached greater trochanter.

Posterior exposure of the hip was the earliest approach described, dating back to Langenbeck in 1874. However this and the later descriptions of Kocher in 1892 and Gibson (1950) involve extensive dissection, which is not appropriate for the minimal exposure necessary for hemiarthroplasty. Moore (1957), in his report on the use of the prosthesis that bears his name, described a more limited posterior exposure – the Southern approach. Tissue dissection, in particular disruption of the abductors, is kept to a minimum and this approach is therefore more appropriate for hip fracture surgery.

Anterior or posterior approach

Papers discussing the choice of approach for hip fracture surgery generally compare an anterior with a posterior approach. The terms here refer to the capsule incision, so an anterior approach generally refers to a lateral, transgluteal or Hardinge approach with an anterior capsular incision. This is therefore a distortion of a true anterior approach and should be avoided if possible. A posterior approach invariably relates to a Moore Southern approach.

Conflicting claims are made regarding the risks and benefits of each approach. Neither can be said to be the best, but the pros and cons are summed up in Table 8.1.

Each method therefore has its own advantages and disadvantages and each surgeon must choose the approach which produces the best results in their hands. The decision will also be influenced by the type of prosthesis to be used. For example, a long-stemmed prosthesis will be easier to insert by a posterior approach, whilst the lack of rotational stability with an uncemented Thompson prosthesis means that a posterior approach should not be used.

The most commonly used approaches of the direct lateral and posterior approach are described here in detail.

Table 8.1

Anterolateral (anterior) approaches

Advantages

Lower risk of dislocation

Possibly lower risk of infection

Disadvantages

Greater tissue dissection

Risk of abductor damage

More restricted access for straight or long stem arthroplasty

Possibly higher risk of venous thrombosis

Posterior approach

Advantages

Limited tissue dissection gives shorter operation times and less blood loss

Possibly lower risk of venous thrombosis

Abductors not dysfunctioned

Lower risk of femoral penetration

Disadvantages

Higher risk of dislocation

Risk of sciatic nerve damage

Possibly higher risk of infection

Operative technique

Positioning of the patient

For an anterolateral approach the operation can be undertaken with the patient supine or in the full lateral position. For a posterior approach the patient must be in the full lateral position. For a supine position the patient is placed with the greater trochanter of the operated side at the very edge of the table, allowing part of the buttock to hang down over the edge. A sandbag is placed under the buttock on the injured side.

For the lateral position the patient is secured on the operating table with a posterior back support and a post anteriorly (Fig. 8.4). The anterior post must be positioned to support the pelvis, but allow for the injured leg to

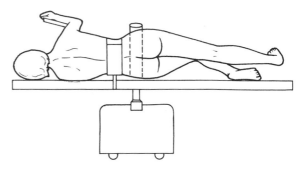

Fig. 8.4 Positioning of the patient in the full lateral position.

be flexed to 90° and then adducted during the operation. It is important that the surgeon checks that the patient is correctly and securely positioned before scrubbing up.

Skin preparation and towelling

The hip is cleansed with an antiseptic solution and draped to allow free movement of the leg. Particular attention to detail is required at this stage to maintain sterility of the operative field. The use of a sterile perineal isolation drape and a clear plastic adhesive dressing over the wound is recommended. If an anterolateral approach is to be used with the patient in the full lateral position, the lower leg will need to be double- or even triple-wrapped as sterility of the foot cannot be guaranteed when the leg is abducted and flexed over the side of the operating table.

Anterolateral approach to the hip

This is also termed the lateral, Hardinge or transgluteal approach. The term anterior refers to the anterior incision into the hip joint capsule. The incision is centred on the greater trochanter with half above and half below. It is either straight or may curve a little posteriorly proximally. The distal half extends in the line of the femur (Fig. 8.5). The exact length of the incision will depend on the ease of exposure, being longer in the more obese or muscular the patient.

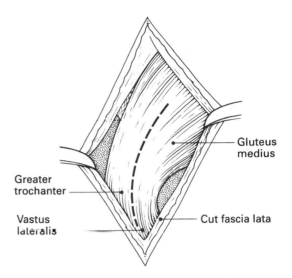

Fig. 8.6 Tensor fascia lata is split longitudinally to reveal the gluteus medius muscles and vastus lateralis, which are split.

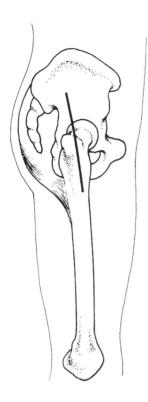

Fig. 8.5 Incision for anterior approach to the hip.

Once through the skin, the iliotibial tract and gluteal fascia more proximally are divided in the line of the incision. Separate any adherent fibres of gluteus medius from the fascia. Any bursal tissue over the greater trochanter is swept away to expose the curved insertion of the gluteus medius into the greater trochanter, which is in the centre of the wound (Fig. 8.6).

The anterior portion of the tendon of gluteus medius is detached from the trochanter, leaving a cuff of tissue for reattachment. The incision extends from the anterior portion of the vastus lateralis, around the trochanter to the apex. At this point the incision runs in the line of the muscle fibres, thus preserving the attachment of the posterior tendinous edge of gluteus medius (Fig. 8.7). The superior gluteal nerve may be injured by excessive incision proximally into gluteus medius. The nerve enters the posterior border of the muscle and fans out in an arc. Any intramuscular incision

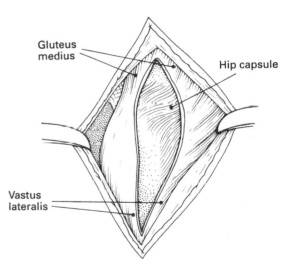

Fig. 8.7 Incision of gluteus medius and vastus lateralis to reveal the anterior joint capsule.

should not extend more than 5 cm from the greater trochanter to be sure of not damaging the nerve. Distally the splitting of the anterior fibres of vastus lateralis can cause troublesome bleeding from branches of the lateral circumflex femoral artery. This can usually be controlled by diathermy.

The femur can now be adducted and externally rotated to bring the anterior capsule into

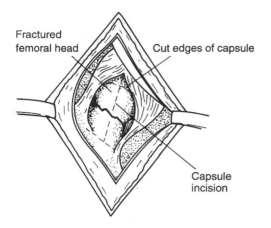

Fractured femoral head

Cut edges of capsule

Capsule incision

Fig. 8.8 The anterior joint capsule is exposed and a T-shaped incision made into it.

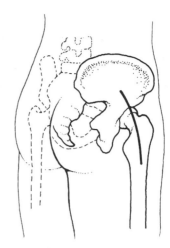

Fig. 8.10 Incision for posterior approach.

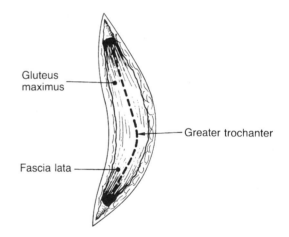

Gluteus maximus

Greater trochanter

Fascia lata

Fig. 8.11 Incision of fascia lata and fibres of gluteus maximus proximally.

view. Gluteus minimus and further fibres of vastus lateralis are cleared away to reveal the iliofemoral ligament and the anterior hip joint capsule, which is incised with an inverted T-shaped incision to open the joint (Fig. 8.8). The upper part of the T is along the inter-trochanteric line, whilst the medial part should extend to the rim of the acetabulum. Haematoma from within the joint capsule will be encountered as the capsule is incised.

Adduction and externally rotating the leg will bring the fracture into view. The hip should be flexed to 90°, fully adducted and externally rotated so that the leg hangs over the side of the operation table and the knee flexes to 90° (Fig. 8.9). An assistant is required to hold the leg in this position.

The femoral neck is exposed to allow it to be cut and the prosthesis inserted as described later in this chapter.

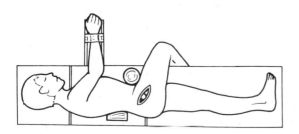

Fig. 8.9 Flexion, abduction and external rotation of the leg reveal the fracture.

Posterior or Southern approach to the hip

Moore's southern approach is performed with the patient in the lateral position, the injured hip uppermost (Fig. 8.4). As for an anterior approach, the hip must be prepared and draped to allow free movement of the injured leg. The incision begins 5 cm distal to the posterior inferior spine and curves down to the posterior edge of the greater trochanter, from where it runs straight down a further 10 cm (Fig. 8.10).

The fascia lata is incised longitudinally and the gluteus maximus inserting into the fascia is split in the line of the fibres (Fig. 8.11). Any bursa tissue is swept away and the short external rotators, piriformis, gemelli, obturator internus and quadratus femoris are displayed (Fig. 8.12).

The sciatic nerve running medially to the femur is protected from injury by dividing the short rotators close to the posterior edge of the trochanter and reflecting the muscles over the nerve with stay sutures (Fig. 8.13).

The gemelli and obturator internus are always divided. The piriformis usually has to be divided, but the lowermost muscle, quadratus femoris, can often be preserved or only partially cut. The quadratus femoris muscle usually has large vessels within it which can

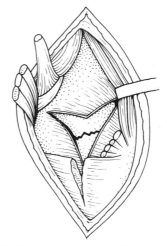

Fig. 8.14   Incision into the capsule.

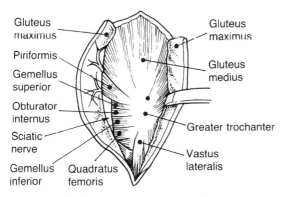

Fig. 8.12   The short rotators are isolated with the sciatic nerve medially.

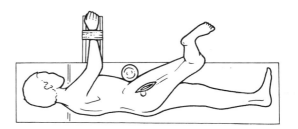

Fig. 8.15   The leg is fully internally rotated and the knee flexed to 90° for cutting the femoral neck.

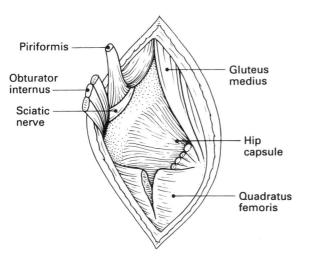

Fig. 8.13   The short rotators are divided close to the femur and used to protect the sciatic nerve.

cause troublesome bleeding. It is best therefore to avoid incising this muscle, unless it is essential to obtain adequate exposure.

Beneath the short rotators is the posterior capsule of the hip, which is opened with a T-shaped incision, the horizontal limb of which is placed parallel to the rim of the acetabulum (Fig. 8.14). The upper part of the T should extend to the acetabular margin. Joint haematoma is aspirated and the capsule reflected to allow access to the joint and the fracture. The femoral neck is exposed to allow access for cutting the femoral neck. The assistant holds the leg fully internally rotated with the knee flexed to 90°. The vertical tibia provides a good guide for checking the alignment of the neck cut and the prosthesis (Fig. 8.15).

Cutting the femoral neck

Regardless of the surgical approach to the hip, the femoral neck will need to be cut at an angle appropriate for the prosthesis to be used. Prior to commencing the cut, ensure that the knee is flexed to 90° and that the tibia is vertical to the floor. The neck is best cut with an oscillating saw. An alternative is a Gigli saw. An osteotome should never be used as this may fracture the femur.

Anterolateral approach

For an anterolateral approach the foot is held down to the floor, with the tibia vertical. The femoral neck cut is then cut from an anterior to posterior direction. The oscillating saw is held vertically and then positioned 5–10° from the vertical, that is, the tip of the saw blade is pointing slightly medially (Fig. 8.16). The anterior angulation of the cut into the femoral head is because the femoral neck normally has 10° of anteversion.

Posterior approach

For a posterior approach the foot is held up and the femoral neck is cut from posterior to

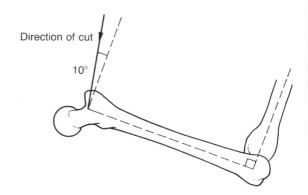

Fig. 8.17   Direction of cut for a posterior approach.

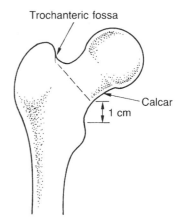

Fig. 8.18   Direction of cut of the femoral neck as viewed from the front for a Moore prosthesis.

anterior. The vertical tibia gives the angulation of cut for the femur, which is 10–15° from the vertical, that is, the tip of the saw blade is pointing slightly laterally (Fig. 8.17).

The approach to the hip will determine the angle of cut of the femoral neck in one plane, and the exact site of the cut angulation in the other plane will be determined by the type of prosthesis to be used.

Moore prosthesis

The cut should extend from the trochanteric fossa laterally to the calcar medially. The calcar should be cut approximately 1–1.5 cm proximal to the upper border of the lesser trochanter (Fig. 8.18). Orientation of the cut

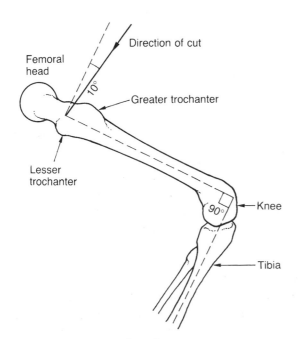

Fig. 8.16   Direction of cut for an anterior approach.

may be aided by aligning a Moore prosthesis parallel to the long axis of the femur.

Thompson prosthesis

The cut should run along the intertrochanteric line, that is, from the trochanteric fossa laterally to the base of the calcar just above the lesser trochanter (Fig. 8.19).

Cemented prosthesis

The direction of cut is the same as for a Thompson prosthesis (Fig. 8.19).

Extracting the femoral head

The femoral head is removed with the aid of a corkscrew inserted into the centre of the femoral head. The corkscrew should be inserted to a sufficient depth and in the middle of the head to enable a good hold to be established. Care needs to be taken not to allow the sharp tip of the corkscrew to penetrate out of the head and damage the acetabular articular surface. Soft tissues attached to the femoral head need to be cut away. The ligament of teres is usually torn when extracting the head, but may need to be cut.

Once the head is extracted the acetabulum should be inspected for wear or damage. Any loose bony debris or soft tissue should be removed and the ligament teres resected if

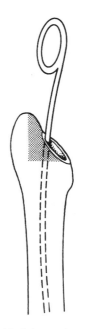

Fig. 8.20 A box chisel is used to remove the shaded area of cancellous bone. A bone spike is then used to define the medullary cavity.

necessary. The size of the femoral head should be measured using a set of semicircular templates of differing sizes. Measuring callipers may be used but they are less accurate. The prosthesis size chosen should not differ by more than 1 mm from that of the head extracted.

Preparing the femur

Excessive force used to prepare the femur may result in a fracture of the femoral shaft. The osteoporotic bone of a hip fracture patient is much weaker than an arthritic patient having a total hip replacement. Ideally the femur should be prepared using only hand-held reamers without the use of a hammer. Occasionally a hammer may be used to complete the preparation, but then only with small gentle taps.

Uncemented Moore prosthesis

A box chisel and hammer are used to remove cancellous bone from the lateral part of the femur (Fig. 8.20). The bone removed can be kept and later used for bone grafting into the

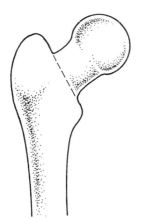

Fig. 8.19 Direction of cut of the femoral neck as viewed from the front for a Thompson or cemented prosthesis.

holes in the prosthesis stem. A bone spike is then inserted by hand into the medullary cavity to a depth of 12 cm in order to define the direction of the canal. The entry point for the spike should be slightly lateral to the middle of the femur. The bone spike should be used to feel a path down the medullary cavity, and excessive force should be avoided as this may push the spike out of the femur.

Reaming of the femur can now be undertaken using hand reamers of appropriate type for the prosthesis being used. The Moore prosthesis is made with a straight or curved stem of standard or narrow sizes. Ideally, reaming should be done entirely by hand. Reaming should concentrate on removing bone from the areas shown in Figure 8.21, as this allows the prosthesis to be inserted in a correct position. Reaming should be undertaken whilst the tibia is held vertical and with 5–15° of anteversion, to match the anteversion of the cut femoral neck.

Uncemented Thompson prosthesis

Because of the smaller stem size, only minimal preparation of the femur is required. For most

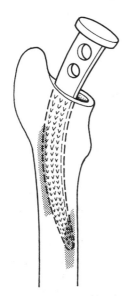

Fig. 8.21 Reaming of the femur should be done by hand if possible. The tibia should be kept vertical and reaming performed with approximately 10° of anteversion to match the cut on the femoral neck. Reaming should concentrate on removing bone in the shaded areas.

cases passing a bone spike down the femur for 12 cm is all that is needed. Occasionally minimal reaming with a small curved reamer may be used. As for a Moore prosthesis, the initial entry point into the medullary cavity should be slightly laterally.

Cemented prosthesis

The medullary cavity should first be defined with a bone spike as for an uncemented prosthesis. The initial entry point into the medullary cavity should be slightly lateral of centre. The extent of reaming will be determined by the size and type of stem to be used. Ideally the reamers should be matched to both the prosthesis and the size of the medullary cavity. Three different stem sizes will normally suffice.

Insertion of the prosthesis

Uncemented prosthesis

Following reaming of the femur a prosthesis of appropriate head size to match the one extracted and of a stem size to match the reamers is gently hammered into place. Remember to keep the tibia vertical and insert the prosthesis with the same degree (usually 10°) of anteversion used for cutting the femoral neck and reaming. With the Moore prosthesis, pieces of medullary bone taken from the femoral head may be placed into the holes in the stem. Excessive force should not be used to hammer the prosthesis into place as this may split the femur. If the prosthesis feels tight and cannot be hammered into position with gentle taps, it should be removed and further reaming of the femur undertaken.

The prosthesis should be inserted so that the collar fits snugly on to the calcar (Fig. 8.22). Occasionally the prosthesis may have to be removed and the neck re-cut with an oscillating saw to achieve this. If reaming of the femur has been correctly performed the prosthesis should also be in a valgus position as opposed to an incorrect varus position.

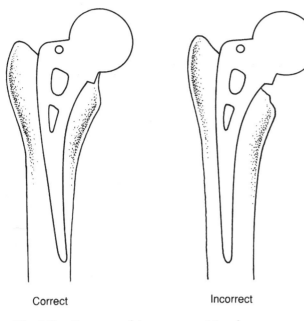

Correct   Incorrect

Fig. 8.22 Correct and incorrect position for an uncemented prosthesis. The collar of the prosthesis should fit comfortably on to the cut calcar. In addition the tip of the stem touches the medial femoral cortex.

Cemented prosthesis

If the prosthesis is to be cemented in place then modern cementing methods should be used. This includes:

1 The femur should have been prepared with reamers that match both the prosthesis stem and the size of the femoral canal. This is to ensure an even cement mantel all around the prosthesis.
2 Use of a cement restrictor. This may either consist of a cylinder of bone taken from the extracted femoral head or a plastic cement restrictor. It should be placed within the medullary cavity at a level just distal to the tip of the prosthesis.
3 The femur is irrigated with saline under pressure to remove debris and marrow tissue. All blood and other debris should be carefully removed from any area in which cement is to be used.
4 Prior to inserting the cement the prosthesis or a similar trial stem and head should be inserted and a trial reduction performed.

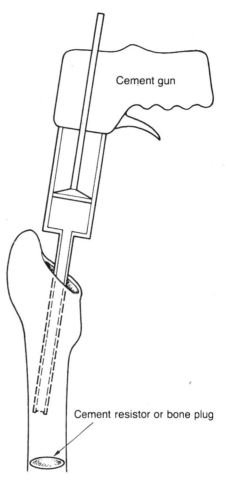

Cement gun

Cement resistor or bone plug

Fig. 8.23 A cement gun should be used to achieve pressurized filling of the canal.

5 The anaesthetist should be informed immediately prior to insertion of cement. There is a risk of cardiac arrhythmias, including ventricular fibrillation, being precipitated by inserting the cement.
6 A venting catheter should be used to allow the air to escape from the femur as the cement is inserted.
7 Cement is inserted into the femur using a cement gun to ensure an uniform pressurized column of cement (Fig. 8.23).
8 Surgeons are advised to familiarize themselves with the setting characteristics of the cement they use. In warm conditions the time to setting will be shorter, but can be prolonged by keeping the cement in the fridge until required.

9 The prosthesis should be inserted into the centre of the cement and pushed firmly into the femur.
10 Pressure should be kept on the cement as it extrudes from around the neck of the femur. Excess cement should be trimmed before it becomes too hard. Ensure that no fragments are left to hinder joint movement or become detached and remain within the acetabulum.

Reduction of the prosthesis

Anterolateral approach

Extend the knee to bring the leg level with the table. Ensure that the lower part of the leg is still sterile. The leg may have been hanging below the level of the towels. It is best to have previously double-wrapped the leg and to discard the outer layer. If a trial reduction has been performed it may even be necessary to have triple-wrapped the leg.

Traction is now applied by an assistant along the line of the femur with the knee slightly flexed. The hip joint position should be approximately 40° of flexion and external rotation. The surgeon then guides the head of the prosthesis towards the empty acetabulum, and with internal rotation the prosthesis is reduced. Care needs to be taken not to forcibly internally rotate the leg as this may result in a fracture of the femoral shaft. Following reduction, check that the hip has a satisfactory range of movement and is stable within reasonable limits (flexion to 90°, 30° internal and external rotation).

Posterior approach

With the knee flexed, traction is applied to the femur to bring the femoral head to the same level as the acetabulum. Only then is external rotation applied to reduce the prosthesis.

Irreducible femoral head

Reduction of the femoral head should be accomplished without undue force. The commonest reason for any difficulty in locating the femoral head in the socket is failure to resect enough femoral neck. If it not possible to reduce the femoral head, consider the following points:

1 Is the femoral head the correct size? A trial reduction of the chosen head can be carried out before the stem is inserted. The head should feel firm, but not tight. The grip should be sufficient to allow the stem to stand upright.
2 Check that there is no obstruction within the acetabulum, such as retained cement or bone fragments.
3 Check that the capsular incision is of sufficient size to allow reduction.
4 Look for the capsule and check that it has not become enfolded and trapped within the joint. This will result in an unstable hip with lack of full extension.
5 Is the prosthesis inserted too proximally such that it would lengthen the leg? Check the calcar length and compare the length of the limb with the contralateral one felt through the towelling. In addition the centre of the prosthesis head should be level with the tip of the greater trochanter. If cement has not been used extract the prosthesis and revise the neck cut to a more distal position. If the prosthesis has been cemented, an extended soft-tissue release will be necessary, with the whole capsule being divided circumferentially. If necessary the psoas tendon can be divided.

Intraoperative femoral fracture

This is a preventable complication, most likely to occur at one of three stages in the operation:

1 Reaming of the femur. Excessive or too vigorous use of the hammer may fracture the femur. The brittle osteoporotic femur of a hip fracture patient will not stand the hammering of reamers that is frequently carried out during arthroplasty for an osteoarthritic hip.
2 Insertion of the prosthesis. This may be

caused by using excessive force due to inadequate reaming of the femur. The stem sizes of the Moore prosthesis vary in thickness from the different manufacturers and each prosthesis should be matched to its appropriate reamers. Pushing the tip of the prosthesis laterally as it is inserted should be avoided as it may perforate the lateral femoral cortex.

3 Reduction of the prosthesis by forcibly internally rotating (for an anterolateral approach) or externally rotating (for a posterior approach). Always ensure that the femoral head is at the level of the acetabulum before gently rotating the limb.

If the fracture is recognized during the operation, it must be exposed, reduced and secured by the most effect method available. This is generally best achieved by splitting the vastus lateralis in the line of its fibres. If this is performed close to its posterior insertion, bleeding can be kept to a minimum.

The pattern and extent of the fracture must be determined. The Whittaker classification (Fig. 8.24) is helpful:

1 *Type 1*: greater trochanter only. This is the least serious and generally does not require any specific fixation.
2 *Type 2*: fracture of the femoral shaft around the implant. This is generally best treated with cerclage wiring. The prosthesis should then be cemented in place, especially if the weight-bearing calcar was fractured.
3 *Type 3*: fracture beneath the tip of the prosthesis. This is the least common type and the hardest to treat generally, necessitating insertion of a longer stem component. Concerns about the fitness of the patient to survive such extended surgery lead some surgeons to consider conservative management of this type of fracture.

Closure of the wound

Regardless of the type of surgical approach, the capsule should have been retained. Repair

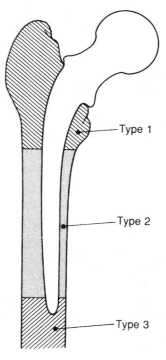

Fig. 8.24 Classification of fractures around implants (see text for details).

of this strong structure will reduce the risk of dislocation. The T-shaped incision through the capsule should be repaired with a strong absorbable suture. The lower part of the T should be fixed to the femur with two or three sutures which may need to be passed through the bone (Fig. 8.25).

If an anterolateral approach was used, the anterior part of the gluteus medius muscle will

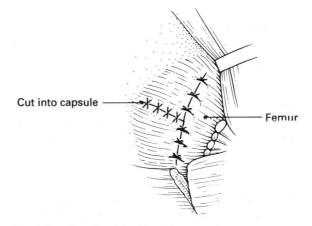

Fig. 8.25 Repair of the hip joint capsule.

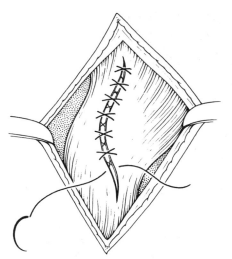

Fig. 8.26   Repair of the gluteus medius muscle following an anterior approach.

have retracted medially and will need to be pulled back to its original insertion as it is sutured back into place (Fig. 8.26). Again, small holes may need to be made into the femur with a bone awl to obtain sufficient hold, or frequently in osteoporotic bone the suture needle may be passed directly through the bone. If a posterior approach was used then the short rotators are reattached to the femur using the stay suture which was used to retract them medially.

The split fascia lata is repaired with a heavy absorbable suture. A fat stitch is only required in the obese. Next the skin edges should be carefully and accurately approximated. Postoperative contamination of the wound frequently occurs in confused elderly hip fracture patients and for this reason it is important to encourage skin healing as soon as possible. The presence of foreign material such as sutures or clips puncturing the skin provides a tract for bacteria to enter and contaminate the wound. The use of a continuous absorbable subcuticular suture is therefore recommended.

Use of drains

Debate continues as to whether a closed suction drain should be used. The value of a drain is to reduce the risk of haematoma formation.

Possible disadvantages are from the risk of sepsis by organisms contaminating the tract of the drain. Blood loss following a hemiarthroplasty should not be excessive as the tissue planes are relatively avascular. It is probably acceptable to drain only those wounds in which blood loss has been excessive.

Postoperative care after arthroplasty

Weight-bearing and mobilization

Following surgery the aim should be to mobilize all patients as soon as possible. Ideally, therefore, patients should begin to mobilize the day after surgery. Prolonged periods of bed rest should be avoided. There should not be any restriction on weight-bearing following an uncomplicated arthroplasty, regardless as to whether cement has been used.

Restriction on hip movement

There is insufficient evidence to suggest that postoperative measures to restrict hip movements will prevent dislocation. The correctly inserted prosthesis seldom dislocates. Therefore there should be no restriction on hip movements.

Check X-ray

An X-ray of the prosthesis is normally taken in the postoperative period (Fig. 8.27). Essential features to note are:

1 No sign of operative fracture of the femur.
2 The head of the arthroplasty is congruent with that of the acetabulum, indicating that a correctly sized prosthesis has been used and that there is no tissue within the joint.
3 The centre of the prosthetic head should be level with the tip of the greater trochanter, indicating that the leg length is correct.

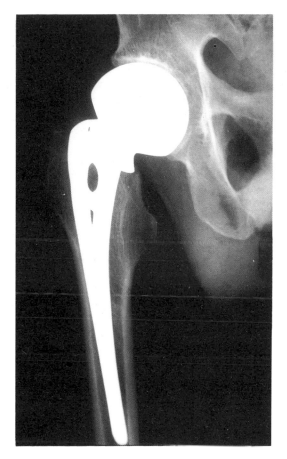

Fig. 8.27 Postoperative check X-ray of an uncemented hemiarthroplasty.

4 If an uncemented prosthesis was used, the tip of the prosthesis should be touching the medial femoral cortex and the collar of the prosthesis should be touching the calcar.

5 For a cemented arthroplasty there should be an even cement mantle of 2–4 mm around the entire length of the prosthesis, with no defects within the cement. The distal tip of the prosthesis should be in the centre of the femoral canal.

Follow-up

Normally outpatient follow-up is arranged to confirm wound healing and check that the hip is functioning satisfactorily. No routine radiological follow-up is indicated. Further intervention is only required if the hip becomes

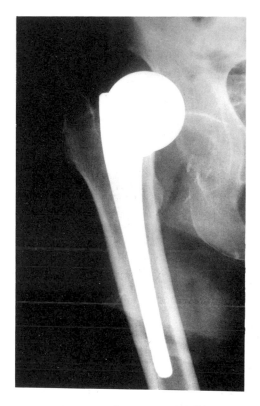

Fig. 8.28 Dislocation of a Moore prosthesis.

sufficiently symptomatic, so long-term follow-up is not routinely indicated.

Complications of arthroplasty

Dislocation

The most common early complication after arthroplasty is dislocation, with an incidence of 2–4%. The diagnosis is usually apparent clinically and is confirmed by X-ray (Fig. 8.28). The prosthesis should be reduced as soon as possible, to relieve pain, but also to prevent damage to adjacent neurovascular structures. The sciatic nerve is particularly vulnerable following posterior dislocation.

Closed reduction should be attempted under general anaesthetic with good muscle relaxation. Inadequate relaxation will risk fracture around the prosthesis. Reduction is best performed with the aid of image intensification. A prosthesis inserted via the posterior approach will dislocate posteriorly and is

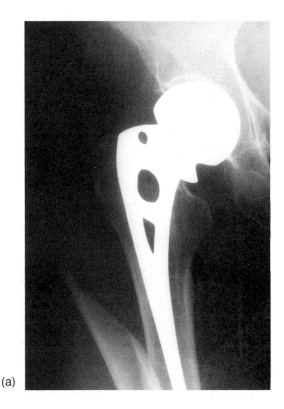
(a)

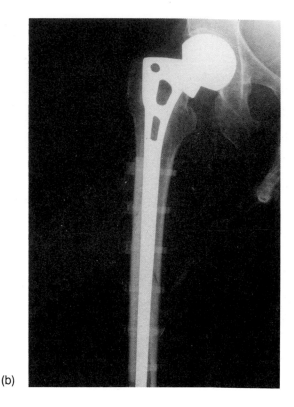
(b)

Fig. 8.29 (a, b) Fracture around a Moore prosthesis treated by conversion to a long stem prosthesis with supplementary Partridge straps.

reduced by longitudinal traction, flexion and external rotation. A prosthesis inserted through an anterolateral approach usually dislocates anteriorly and is reduced by longitudinal traction, flexion and internal rotation. However if it has been inserted in retroversion it may dislocate posteriorly. Once reduced, the stability of the prosthesis should be assessed using the image intensifier to determine for which position and rotation of the hip dislocation occurs.

Bipolar prostheses may be difficult to reduce by closed means. The mobile head should be visualized with X-ray screening to allow the leg to be positioned in the most favourable alignment. Closed reduction will not be possible for a bipolar arthroplasty in which the prosthetic head has become separated from the stem. The surgeon should therefore be prepared to perform an open reduction with a dislocated bipolar prosthesis.

If the dislocation occurs within days of the operation and the prosthesis appears stable when screened at reduction, there is little point in confining the patient to bed for a number of weeks. If the dislocation occurs some weeks later, a period in bed to allow soft-tissue healing may be appropriate. However, this should be kept to a minimum; a more acceptable method is the application of a hip hinge cast brace to restrict movement at the hip. Unfortunately, this may be poorly tolerated by an elderly patient. An alternative if the hip is only dislocated in flexion is to apply a plaster cylinder to the leg. This will limit hip flexion whilst permitting mobilization.

Recurrent dislocation should be treated by revision of the prosthesis, unless the patient is unfit for surgery and already immobile. The longer the procedure is delayed and the more times the prosthesis dislocates, the less likely the patient is to regain pre-injury levels of independence and mobility. The reason for the instability should be identified preoperatively if possible, to assist planning of the surgery. The prosthesis may be tight, or excessively loose. The acetabulum may be damaged or have something lodged within it. If the prosthesis is uncemented, rotational instability is the most likely cause and can be corrected by cementing the prosthesis in the correct alignment. A cemented prosthesis will be more difficult to revise and should not be undertaken unless the surgeon is skilled in revision arthroplasty. Removal of the well-fixed cement from an osteoporotic femoral shaft runs a considerable risk of fracturing the shaft.

Unfortunately, after dislocation the mortality and morbidity are significantly increased to in excess of 50%. Wound and chest infection or thromboembolic complications are the main complications.

Fracture around the prosthesis

Fracture around the femoral stem may only become apparent postoperatively. Increasing pain, the inability to weight-bear, or external rotation of the leg, should alert the doctor to the possibility of a fracture. This may be difficult to identify on X-ray and a clear lateral view is essential, in addition to the AP film.

Fractures in the region of the greater trochanter may be treated conservatively. Those involving the calcar area usually cause persistent pain and revision surgery is the best option. More extensive fractures around the implant or at the tip are difficult to treat and frequently require extensive revision surgery (Fig. 8.29).

Prosthesis loosening

An uncemented prosthesis will frequently sink within the femur until the collar is level with the lesser trochanter. In addition the prosthesis often tilts into a varus position (Fig. 8.30). Neither of these changes is diagnostic of loosening or correlates well with pain in the

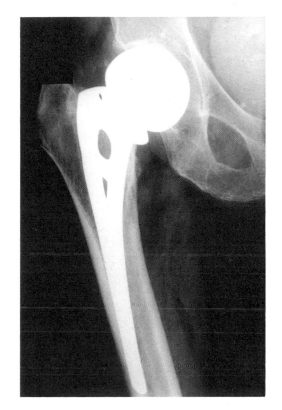

Fig. 8.30 An uncemented prosthesis which has sunk within the femur and tilting into a varus position.

hip. Loosening is seen radiologically as radiolucent lines around the prosthesis, or as erosions which may also occur with sepsis (Fig. 8.31). Loosening is much more common after an uncemented prosthesis and is more likely to be associated with symptoms of pain and reduced mobility.

Pain and disability from a loose implant may rob an elderly patient of their independence. Depending on the patient's physical state and degree of symptoms revision surgery is indicated. The techniques of revision arthroplasty are beyond the scope of this book.

Para-articular calcification

This is also termed heterotopic ossification, and is due to ectopic bone formation within the tissues around the prosthesis (Fig. 8.31).

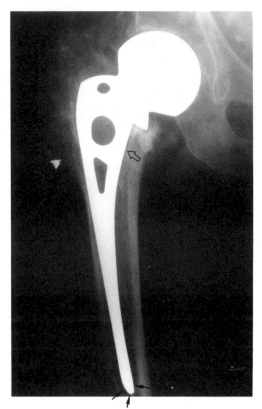

Fig. 8.31 Severe loosening with cavitation around the tip of the prosthesis (small arrows). Radiolucent lines are seen around the collar (open arrow). There is marked para-articular calcification. The additional metal fragment laterally is a remnant of previous internal fixation.

For hip fracture patients it has not been associated with pain or a poor functional result.

Acetabular protrusion

This is a complication which takes some years to occur with a hemiarthroplasty. The reported incidence in long-term survivors is approximately 20%, although many cases are not symptomatic. The incidence may be reduced by using a bipolar prosthesis. Symptoms are of increasing pain and stiffness of the hip and the diagnosis is confirmed by X-ray (Fig. 8.32). Treatment is by revision arthroplasty if symptoms indicate.

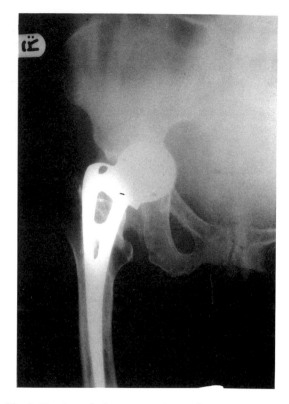

Fig. 8.32 Acetabular protrusion of an uncemented Moore prosthesis.

Key references and further reading

Calder SJ, Anderson GH, Jagger C, Harper WM, Gregg PJ. Unipolar or bipolar prosthesis for displaced intracapsular hip fracture in octogenarians: a randomised prospective trail. *J Bone Joint Surg* 1996; **78**–B:391–394.

Cobb JP. Why use drains? *J Bone Joint Surg* 1990; **72**–B:933–935.

Dall D. Exposure of the hip by anterior osteotomy of the greater trochanter: a modified anterolateral approach. *J Bone Joint Surg* 1986; **68**–B:382–386.

Frndak PA, Mallory TH, Lombardi AV. Translateral surgical approach to the hip; the abduction muscle 'split'. *Clin Orthop* 1993; **295**:135–141.

Hardinge K. The direct lateral approach to the hip. *J Bone Joint Surg* 1982; **64**–B:17–19.

Keene GS, Parker MJ. Hemiarthroplasty of the hip – the anterior or posterior approach? A comparison of surgical approaches. *Injury* 1993; 24:611–613.

Lennox IAC, McLauchlan J. Comparing the mortality and morbidity of cemented and uncemented hemiarthroplasties. *Injury* 1993; **24**:185–186.

McFarland B, Osborne G. Approach to the hip: a suggested improvement on Kocher's method. *J Bone Joint Surg* 1954; **36–B**:364–367.

Moore AT. The self-locking metal hip prosthesis. *J Bone Joint Surg* 1957; **39–A**:811–827.

Pryor GA. A study of the influence of technical adequacy on the clinical result of Moore hemiarthroplasty. *Injury* 1990; **21**:361–365.

Smith-Petersen MN. Approach to and exposure of the hip joint per mold arthroplasty. *J Bone Joint Surg* 1949; **31–A**:40.

Sonne-Holm S, Walter S, Jensen JS. Moore. Hemiarthroplasty with and without bone cement in femoral neck fractures: a clinical controlled trial. *Acta Orthop Scand* 1982; **53**:953–956.

Tronzo RG. *Surgery of the Hip Joint.* Lea & Febiger, Philadelphia, 1973.

Whittaker RP, Sotos LN, Ralston EL. Fractures of the femur about femoral endoprostheses. *J Trauma* 1974; **14**:675–694.

9

Postoperative care

On return from theatre, the hip fracture patient may present a daunting series of different problems for the junior doctor to manage. However, many of these problems can be anticipated, as they are usually a consequence of one or more of the following factors:

1 The patient's preoperative physical and mental state.
2 The fracture type and surgical treatment.
3 The anaesthetic and analgesic drugs used in the perioperative period.

The premorbid status of the patient

There is no substitute for a sound knowledge of the individual patient, or if unfamiliar to the junior doctor, careful assessment of the medical notes made on admission. However, many of the problems likely to become manifest are related to the metabolic and homeostatic dysfunction characteristic of the elderly.

A number of physiological changes occur with ageing that must be considered when managing the elderly patient after hip fracture surgery. Moreover the greater incidence of chronic diseases such as diabetes, hypertension and atherosclerosis may be superimposed on the normal age-related deterioration in organ function. Consequently, multisystem

dysfunction should be considered the norm and postoperative management adjusted accordingly.

Cardiovascular system

Resting cardiac output does not decline with ageing, but increased output is brought about by increasing stroke volume rather than heart rate, as occurs in the young. In practice therefore, volume depletion is poorly tolerated and may place additional strain on an ischaemic heart, expending more energy trying to boost output in the face of declining venous return.

Conduction disorders within the heart and reduced elasticity of the arteries also add to the inability of the aged cardiovascular system to respond to perioperative stress. Not surprisingly, half of postoperative deaths in the elderly are related to the cardiovascular system. Great care must therefore be taken to maintain accurate fluid balance, avoiding inadvertent excessive intravenous infusion as well as dehydration.

Clinical assessment is often difficult: patients may be dehydrated on admission or, more commonly, made so while waiting for surgery. However, the physical signs of skin turgor and dry tongue are less reliable in the elderly. Urinary catheterization may occasionally be required to monitor fluid output.

Respiratory system

The chest wall becomes less expansile with ageing and the kyphotic deformity resulting from multiple osteoporotic vertebral collapse leads to reduced rib excursion. In combination with decreased lung compliance, this produces an increased residual volume and greater dead space. As a result any respiratory depression, caused by anaesthetic agents, narcotic analgesics or sedatives, will produce greater hypoxia than in a young patient. Arterial PO_2 declines with age and therefore postoperative hypoxia is virtually inevitable.

In consequence, these patients should all be given oxygen by mask for at least 24 h after the operation and for the next 3 nights. The aim should be to prevent the typical picture, usually developing at night, of an elderly hypoxic patient becoming increasingly confused, being sedated and becoming more hypoxic as a result.

Renal function

Renal cortical mass declines with age, resulting in a linear reduction in glomerular filtration rate after the age of 40 years. This reduction makes the elderly more vulnerable to acute renal failure after hypotensive episodes.

Renal tubular function is also reduced in the elderly patient, making the aged kidney less efficient at dealing with electrolyte or fluid overload. The functioning of the renin–angiotensin system is also impaired, making sodium and water retention in response to reduced intravascular volume less effective.

In practice these changes make maintenance of fluid balance in the elderly very difficult. The margin between dehydration and overload is small. Excessive saline infusion easily precipitates congestive cardiac failure, while fluid depletion may occur insidiously. The elderly may be reluctant to drink, or take only water, leading to progressive hyponatraemia.

Suggested perioperative care

Before going on to discuss specific complications, the recommended management of the uncomplicated case is presented here:

1 The operation should have taken place within 24 h of admission, on a planned trauma list, in normal working hours.
2 Whether regional or general anaesthetic has been given, in the immediate postoperative period the patient should be awake, breathing spontaneously with the use of supplementary oxygen.
3 The patient should return to the ward in daylight when adequate staff are on duty to monitor him or her carefully and provide reassurance. Nurses should be alert to the potential complications, checking conscious level, respiration, pulse and blood pressure, wound drainage and undertaking pressure-area care.
4 Adequate analgesia should have been given. If regional anaesthesia has been used, sufficient analgesia should be given to ensure that pain relief is maintained. Patient-controlled analgesia is the ideal, allowing the patient to vary opiate injection according to pain level. However it requires an alert patient: many elderly people may be unable to cope with its use. Furthermore, respiratory depression and hypoxia can still occur. Opiate requirements can be reduced by the use of non-steroidal anti-inflammatory drugs which may be given rectally as the intramuscular route is painful. However gastrointestinal bleeding with non-steroidal drugs is more likely in the elderly. Moreover these drugs may potentiate the effects of low-dose heparin and aggravate renal failure.
5 Heightened anxiety can increase pain perception; in the elderly sympathetic surroundings and nursing are important. Reassurance and clear explanations are particularly helpful to calm the elderly

patient who wakes in strange unfamiliar surroundings.

6 Nurses should be confident to turn patients regularly, preventing pressure sores developing. Use of the various pressure sore risk scores is of limited value in these patients, since all must be considered at high risk of pressure sores. The most critical times are while on the emergency room trolley and in the operating theatre. Postoperatively the risk of pressure sores is ever-present. A combination of pressure, shearing forces and friction produces damage to blood vessels and hence ischaemic changes within the skin. The damage is exacerbated by moisture causing maceration of the skin and further harm occurs with wet sheets rubbing or sticking to the skin.

7 Elderly hip fracture patients are especially vulnerable to pressure ulceration because of their often poor nutritional status, low haemoglobin and less resilient skin. The surgeon must permit whatever measures are required for appropriate nursing care and early mobilization. With very few exceptions, the postoperative instructions from the operating surgeon should state: 'mobilize without restrictions'. It is essential that the surgeon recognizes that restoration of the patient's confidence is paramount. The surgeon's instructions must impart confidence to the nurses, who in turn can reassure the patient that everything has gone well.

Initial management

The junior doctor reviewing the patient in the first 24 h after surgery should assess the following:

1 *Respiration* – adequate depth and rate. Is the patient tolerating the oxygen mask? Respiratory depression due to opiates must be reversed with naloxone. Retained secretions and atelectasis, common after long operations, should be treated by vigorous physiotherapy, providing the patient can cooperate.

2 *Mental state* – is the patient restless? If so, is this due to hypoxia, pain, a full bladder? Cautious sedation should only be given when other treatable causes have been excluded. When night sedation is necessary, chloral hydrate, dichloralphenazone or chlormethiazole can be given. The benzodiazepines should be avoided in the elderly.

3 *Cardiovascular system* – assessment of clinical signs includes pulse, its rate, rhythm and volume, blood pressure and peripheral perfusion. The patient may be breathless through cardiac or pulmonary pathology. In the former, other signs of cardiac failure will be evident, such as raised jugular venous pressure, pink frothy sputum, dependent oedema and irregular pulse. The electrocardiogram should be compared with the preoperative tracing and the chest X-ray will reveal a large heart and signs of congestion in the lungs. Myocardial infarction may be painless, especially in the elderly.

4 *Fluid balance* – in hypovolaemia, it is essential to distinguish between fluid depletion and redistribution. The duration of preoperative fluid deprivation is important – was the patient starved then cancelled once or more? Was an intravenous infusion commenced preoperatively? It should be possible to estimate likely blood loss: an intracapsular fracture leads to relatively little blood loss, limited by the capsule and small area of bone exposed. Moreover if internal fixation has been performed there will be no need to suspect significant blood loss.

In contrast, open reduction and internal fixation of a comminuted extracapsular fracture will produce substantial blood loss. Bleeding from the fracture site alone may exceed that from a femoral shaft fracture. Moreover surgery will involve division of vessels within the vastus lateralis, which may lead to further bleeding. The extent of fluid and blood replacement should be calculated and transfusion either commenced or accelerated.

Subsequent management

The day after the operation, the elderly patient should be ready to begin mobilization, in preparation for active rehabilitation. Many of these elderly patients feel that the fracture and subsequent hospitalization spell the end of their independent existence. To be back on their feet, albeit with difficulty and discomfort, within a couple of days of the fall, restores their morale considerably.

In addition to those already discussed, the main complications to be faced in the first week will be thromboembolic and infective. The priorities are to ensure that blood loss has been adequately replaced. Intravenous infusion may then be dispensed with, allowing unhampered mobilization. Similarly, the wound drains, if present, should be removed not later than 48 h postoperatively.

The postoperative X-ray

A check X-ray is performed, if not already carried out in theatre. For internal fixation, the position of the screws or pins within the head is judged. Even if not ideal, unrestricted mobilization is appropriate. There is no evidence to suggest that screws are less likely to cut-out if the patient is confined to bed postoperatively. If the position is judged to be so poor that cut-out is inevitable, then immediate revision is required. For hemiarthroplasty, the technical adequacy of the alignment is judged by assessing head size, neck length, prosthesis stem shaft-angle and calcar seating, as discussed in Chapter 8. The X-ray should also be checked for any periprosthetic fracture.

Postoperative pyrexia

A pyrexia within 24 h of surgery is not necessarily indicative of an infection. However, if it persists, then sepsis is certainly

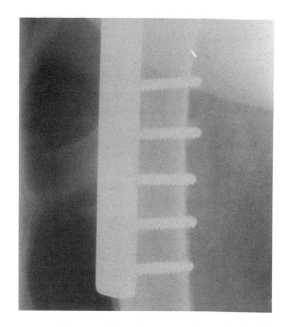

Fig. 9.1 Radiograph of a large abscess around a dynamic hip screw. The fluid extends around the plate.

likely. The main sites to be considered will be the wound, the chest and the urinary tract. Blood, urine and sputum cultures should be taken.

Wound infection

Wound infection is indicated by the classical signs of redness, swelling, pain and temperature. Any discharge should be swabbed for culture and sensitivity before any intravenous antibiotics are commenced. Deep infection around the prosthesis has a delayed presentation some weeks after the original operation. Clinical signs may be non-specific, such as general malaise and increasing pain around the hip. Pyrexia is usually present and the white cell count will be raised. Radiographic signs take some weeks to develop and may be minimal (Figs 9.1 and 9.2). In later stages bone destruction will be evident with radiographic signs of osteomyelitis. Radiographic signs suggestive of sepsis for an arthroplasty are ambiguous but include loss of the joint space from destruction of articular cartilage and radiolucency around the prosthetic stem.

The most likely organisms will be a staphylococcus, streptococcus or the Gram-negative

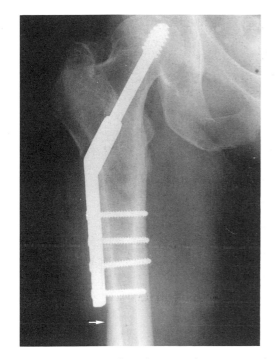

Fig. 9.2 Sepsis around a dynamic hip screw plate. There is erosion of cortical bone around the distal end of the plate (arrow).

organisms common in hospital. The antibiotics prescribed should cover all these possibilities. Deep infection after internal fixation or hemiarthroplasty may require debridement and removal of the implant. The presence of a cemented prosthesis will complicate the picture. The same principles apply as for the management of the infected total hip replacement. These are outside the scope of this book.

Chest infection

In chest and urinary tract infections, Gram-negative organisms must be considered. Postoperative pneumonia is likely to be due to *Streptococcus pneumoniae*, *Haemophilus influenzae* or *Staphylococcus aureus*. A reasonable primary treatment combination would be flucloxacillin and ampicillin.

Urinary tract infection

Urinary tract infections, with systemic upset, are best treated with appropriate broad-spectrum antibiotics, unless sensitivities are available.

Antibiotic-induced diarrhoea

The use of prophylactic antibiotics in implant surgery is well-established and most, if not all, hip fracture patients will receive antibiotics while in hospital. However, if used solely to prevent rather than treat infection, the course should be short – three or four perioperative intravenous doses.

Diarrhoea is a common side-effect of prolonged antibiotic therapy and potentially one of the most serious causes for this is *Clostridium difficile* which is more of a risk in the elderly and infirm. *C. difficile* is normally found in a small proportion of healthy persons and may colonize the gut without any harmful effects. Oral broad-spectrum antibiotics such as ampicillin, cephalosporins or ciprofloxacin are most often the cause of *C. difficile*-associated diarrhoea. Intravenous antibiotic therapy can also produce diarrhoea and prolonged or repeated therapy increases the risk.

The symptoms range from mild to life-threatening, with development of toxic megacolon which may occur in the absence of diarrhoea. In most cases there is watery, foul-smelling diarrhoea and where pseudomembranous colitis develops, fever, abdominal pain and distension occur. Antibiotics may have been stopped by the time the clinical features develop. If not, therapy should be stopped as soon as possible. In its mildest form, no treatment is required. In most cases, however, vancomycin or metronidazole is effective.

Bowel and bladder function

Postoperative urinary retention is more common in the elderly male. The admission history must include features suggestive of prostatic hypertrophy, frequency, nocturia, hesitancy and poor stream. If necessary a catheter should be inserted in theatre prior to operation. This should remain *in situ* until the patient is mobile again. In the post-operative period the doctor should be alert for chronic retention with overflow. Catheterization to determine the residual volume may be useful.

Many elderly patients will be taking regular laxatives prior to admission. Following surgery some degree of constipation is very common, especially in the elderly. The junior doctor is often asked to prescribe a laxative. The possibility of coincidental bowel pathology must be considered and a rectal examination is essential.

The safest and most appropriate laxatives in the elderly are bulk-forming agents, e.g. bran, methylcellulose. Osmotic preparations, e.g. lactulose, magnesium salts, are also useful and can be taken safely for prolonged periods if necessary. Stimulant agents such as bisacodyl and danthron must be reserved for short-term use, if there has been no response to the other measures.

Thromboembolic complications

If routine venography is performed on all hip fracture patients, the incidence of venous thrombosis is approximately 55%. This figure is considerably reduced if thromboembolic prophylactic measures are taken, as discussed in Chapter 3. In clinical practice the incidence of venous thrombosis suspected on clinical grounds and confirmed by investigations is only 3%. This indicates that most thrombi are undetected. The same is true for pulmonary emboli where the reported incidence from clinical reports is approximately 2%.

Some swelling of the leg is a normal finding after a hip fracture and therefore this is not a useful clinical sign of venous thrombosis. However, for a proximal thrombus considerable swelling of the entire leg can occur. Tenderness in the calf is a more helpful sign. The diagnosis of venous thrombosis should always be confirmed by one of a number of available investigations. Ultrasound venography is a quick, safe and reliable method of detecting thrombi within the femoral and popliteal veins. Thrombi distal to the knee are less easily demonstrated by this technique. Contrast venography will demonstrate thrombi within the distal veins, but is more invasive and not without risks. Radioisotope scanning can be used as an alternative.

The treatment for pulmonary emboli and venous thrombi proximal to the knee is therapeutic anticoagulation with heparin and later warfarin. For thrombi distal to the knee the preferred method of treatment is controversial, with some physicians opting for full anticoagulation, whilst others adopt a 'wait-and-see' policy, prescribing anticoagulants only if there are signs of extension or embolization of the thrombosis.

Nutrition

Many elderly patients suffer from nutritional deficiencies, but the problem is even more prevalent with hip fracture patients. This has been documented in numerous studies, as has the fact that supplementary feeding, if necessary using a nasogastric tube, will significantly reduce the incidence of postoperative complications, hospital stay and mortality.

Prevention of further fractures

Despite the increasing incidence of fractures among the elderly there are a few measures that have been proven to reduce the risk of fracture occurring. Methods of preventing further fractures may involve:

1 Increasing the bone strength.
2 Reducing the risk of falling.
3 Reducing the consequences of falling.

Increasing the bone strength

Hormone replacement therapy remains the most useful method of retaining bone stock for women. However, as yet there are no randomized studies to demonstrate its effectiveness in reducing the risk of hip fracture. To be efficacious it should be used within 10 years of the menopause and taken for a minimum of 10 years. Adverse effects are menstrual bleeding and a small increase in the risk of carcinoma of the breast. The beneficial effects on bone stock may be lost when treatment is stopped. Hormone replacement therapy should however be considered in all females who sustain a hip fracture within 10 years of the menopause.

Calcium (1200 mg) and vitamin D (800 units) tablets have been shown in a randomized placebo-controlled trial to reduce the risk of further hip fractures. This treatment should be considered for all patients who sustain a hip fracture. The bisphosphonates calcitriol, calcitonin and fluoride are other drugs which may be of benefit, but further research is required to demonstrate their effectiveness before any firm recommendations can be made for their use following a hip fracture.

Reducing the risk of falling

Physical inactivity is associated with an increased risk of fractures, but as yet it has not been possible to conclusively demonstrate that specific exercise programmes will reduce the risk of hip fractures.

Reducing the consequences of falling

Protective padding around the hip has been shown to reduce the risk of fracturing the hip during falling. However further research is required to determine which patients would benefit from such padding and to assess compliance and effectiveness.

Key references

Chapuy MC, Arlot ME, Delmas PD, Meunier PJ. Effect of calcium and cholecalciferol treatment for three years on hip fractures in elderly women. *Br Med J* 1994; **308**:1081–1082.

Delmi M, Rapin C-H, Bengoa J-M, Delmas PD, Vasey H, Bonjour J-P. Dietary supplementation in elderly patients with fractured neck of femur. *Lancet* 1990; **335**:1013–1016.

Grady-Benson JC, Oishi CS, Hanson PB, Colwell CW, Otis SM, Walker RH. Postoperative surveillance for deep venous thrombosis with duplex ultrasonography after total knee arthroplasty. *J Bone Joint Surg* 1994; **76–A**:1649–1657.

Jensen TT, Juncker Y. Pressure sores common after hip operations. *Acta Orthop Scand* 1987; **58**:209–211.

Lauritzen JB, Petersen MM, Lund B. Effects of external hip protectors on hip fractures. *Lancet* 1993; **341**:11–13.

Parker MJ, Palmer CR. Prediction of rehabilitation after hip fracture. *Age Ageing* 1995; **24**:96–98.

Seymour G. *Medical Assessment of the Elderly Surgical Patient.* Croom Helm, London, 1986.

Seymour DG, Vaz FG. A prospective study of elderly general surgical patients: II. Post-operative complications. *Age Ageing* 1989; **18**:316–326.

Versluysen M. How elderly patients with femoral fracture develop pressure sores in hospital. *Br Med J* 1986; **292**:1311–1313.

Zuckerman JD. *Orthopaedic Injuries in the Elderly.* Urban & Schwarzenberg, Baltimore, MD, 1990.

Index

Acetabular erosion, 20, 130
Aetiology, 2–5
Age:
  bone loss and, 2, 3
  falls and, 2–3, 4
  hip fracture incidence and, 2–3
Anaemia, 31
Anaesthesia, 37
Analgesia, 32–3, 134
Anterolateral approach, 114, 115–16
  cutting of femoral neck, 120
  operative technique, 116–18
  prosthesis reduction, 124
Antibiotic prophylaxis, 35–7
Antibiotic-induced diarrhoea, 137
AO classification system:
  extracapsular fractures, 14, 15, 13–17
  intracapsular fractures, 12–13
AO screws, 53
Approach, *See* Surgical approach
Arthritis of the hip, 22
Arthroplasty:
  choice of prosthesis, 111–12
  complications, 127–30
    acetabular erosion, 120
    dislocation, 127–9
    fracture around prosthesis, 129, 20
    para-articular calcification, 129
    prosthesis loosening, 129
  elderly patients, 19–20
  indications for, 21, 45
  intracapsular fractures, 21–2

Arthroplasty—*cont.*
  operative technique, 116–26
    cutting of femoral neck, 120–1
    extracting the femoral head, 121
    femur preparation, 121–2
    intraoperative femoral fracture, 124–5
    positioning of patient, 116
    prosthesis insertion, 122–3
    prosthesis reduction, 124
    skin preparation, 116
    surgical approach, 113–16
    wound closure, 125–6
  postoperative care, 126–7
  use of cement, 112–13
Asnis screws, 53, 54
Aspiration of the hip, 50
Aspirin, 32, 35
Avascular necrosis
  extracapsular fractures, 87–8
  intracapsular fractures, 60
  radiographic signs, 58

Barthel index, 30
Basal fractures, 15, 78–80
Bipolar prosthesis, 112
Bisphosphonates, 4, 139
Bladder function, 137–8
Bone grafting, 76
Bone loss, 2–4
Bone mineral density, 3

Bone strength, 31
  increasing, 138–9
Bowel function, 137–8

Calcitonin, 4
Calcium supplementation, 4, 139
Cardiac function, 29
  postoperative management, 135
  premorbid status, 133–4
Cement:
  extramedullary fractures, 76
  use in arthroplasty, 112–13, 121, 122, 123
Cervical fractures *see* Intracapsular fractures
Charnley approach, 115
Chest infection, 137
Chronic renal failure, 22
Classification fracture, 10–17
  intracapsular fractures, 11–13
    Garden, 11–12
    Pauwels, 12–13
  extracapsular, 13–17
    Jensen, 14
    AO, 12–13, 14–17
    Fielding, 14
    Zickle, 14
    Seinsheimer, 14
Clostridium difficile, 137
Computed tomography, 9
Conservative treatment, 18, 25–26

Dextran, 35
Deyerle pins, 54
Diagnosis, 2–10
Diarrhoea, antibiotic-induced, 137
Diet *see* Nutrition
Direct lateral approach *see* Anterolateral
    approach
Dislocation
  following arthroplasty, 20, 127–9
Distal lacking of intramedullary nail, 104–6
Drains, use of, 36
  in arthroplasty, 126
Dynamic extramedullary implants, 23
Dynamic hip screw (DHS), 23–5
  complications, 85–9
    avascular necrosis, 87–8
    cut-out, 85–6
    detachment of plate from femur, 86–7
    non-union, 87
  intracapsular fractures, 55–6

Dynamic hip screw—*cont.*
  osteotomy and, 64
  subtrochanteric fractures, 82–4

Ender's nail, 24, 92–3
Evans classification system, 14
Extracapsular fractures, 3–4, 10–11
  basal fractures, 15, 78–80
  classification of, 13–15, 16–17
  reversed fracture line, 81–2
  traction, 24
  see also Extramedullary fixation;
    Intramedullary fixation;
    Subtrochanteric fractures;
    Trochanteric fractures
Extramedullary fixation, 22–4, 63–89
  implant removal, 88
  indications for, 24
  postoperative management, 84–5
  supplementary fixation, 75
  surgical technique, 63–77
    bone grafting, 76
    cement augmentation, 76
    complication
      cut-out, 85–6
      plate detachment, 86–7
      non-union, 87
      avascular necrosis, 87–8
    compression screw use, 74
    guidewire positioning, 66–70
    lag screw insertion, 70–1
    Medoff sliding plate, 76, 77
    short barrel plate use, 75
    side plate application, 71–3
    surgical approach, 65–6
    trochanteric stabilizing plate use, 77
    wound closure, 73–4
  see also Dynamic hip screw; Fracture
    Reduction

Falls, 2
  age-related changes, 2–3, 4
  recurrent, 32
  reducing consequences of, 139
  reducing risk of, 139
  sustained injuries, 29
Fascia lata, 65, 97, 117, 126
Femoral shaft fracture, 24
Fielding and Magliato classification system,
    14

Fluid balance, postoperative management, 135
Fracture classification, 10–17 *see* classification
Fracture reduction
  extracapsalar fractures
    extramedullary fixation, 63–4
    intramedullary fixation, 94–7
  intracapsular fractures
    closed reduction, 46–8
    open reduction, 48–50
Fracture table, 39–44

Gamma nail, 23, 24, 92, 97, 107
Garden alignment index, 48
Garden grading system, 11–13
Garden screws, 50, 53
Gouffon screws, 53
Guidewire positioning:
  extracapsular fractures, extramedullary fixation, 66–70
  intracapsular fractures, internal fixation, 50–5
  extracapsular fractures, intramedullary fixation, 98–9

Hansson hook pins, 50, 54
Hardinge approach, 114–6
Hemiarthroplasty *see* Arthroplasty
Heparin, 34
Hip fracture:
  causes of, 2–5
  classification of, 10–17
  diagnosis, 7–10
  incidence, 1–2
    geographic variation, 1, 2
    racial variation, 1–2
  medical assessment, 29–32
  treatment options, 17–25
  see also individual types of fractures and treatments
Hormone replacement therapy, 4, 138–9
Huckstep nail, 97–8
Hypothermia, 33
Hypovolaemia, 33, 135

Image intensifier, 39–43
Impacted intracapsular fractures, 7–9, 11
Incidence, 1–2

Infection, 20, 31
  chest, 137
  urinary tract, 137
  wound, 136–7
  prophylaxis, 35–7
Internal fixation, intracapsular fracture
  choice of implant, 46
  complications, 57–61
    avascular necrosis, 59, 60
    backing out of the screws, 60
    early re-displacement, 57
    non-union, 58–60
  compression, 56
  indications for, 18–21, 45
  minimally displaced fractures, 18
  osteosynthesis device positioning, 50–6
    dynamic hip screw fixation, 55–6
    three or more screws, 53–5
    two hook pins or screws, 50–3
  postoperative management, 56–7
    follow-up, 57
    hip function, 56
    weight-bearing, 56–7
  timing of surgery, 45–6
  undisplaced fractures, 17, 18
  see also Fracture reduction
Intracapsular fractures,
  classification of, 11–13
  treatment options, 18–21
  see also Arthroplasty; Internal fixation
Intramedullary fixation:
  choice of implant, 91–3
  complications, 107–8
    operative fracture, 107
    later femur fracture, 107
    cut-out, 107
    non-union, 107–8
  indications for, 24–5, 91
  operative technique, 93–107
    distal locking of nail, 104–6
    entry point in femur, 97–8
    femoral lag screw positioning, 101–4
    lag screw insertion, 101–4
    guidewire insertion, 98–9
    incision, 97
    nail insertion, 99–100
    preoperative planning, 93–4
    reaming of femur, 99
    reduction of fracture, 94–7
    wound closure, 106

Intramedullary fixation—*cont.*
  postoperative management, 106–7
Isotope bone scan, 9

Jensen and Michaelsen classification system,
    14–15

Knowles pins, 54
Küntscher-Y nail, 24, 92, 97

Leadbetter manoeuvre, 48

McFarland-Osborne approach, 114–15
Magnetic resonance imaging, 10
Mental state, 30
Metabolic bone disease, 22
Moore prosthesis, 120, 121–3
Moore Southern approach, 115, 118

Non-treatment, 25–6
Non-union:
  intracapsular fractures, 19, 58–60
  extracapsular fractures, 87, 107–8
Nutrition, 31, 138

Open reduction:
  extracapsular fractures, 64
  intracapsular fractures, 48–50
Osteomalacia, 4
Osteotomy, 64

Paget's disease, 22, 31
Para-articular calcification, 129–30
Parkinson's disease, 30
Pathological fractures, 22, 25, 31
Pauwels classification system, 12
Pertrochanteric fractures, 15, 83
Posterior approach, 115–16
  cutting of femoral neck, 120
  operative technique, 118–19
  prosthesis reduction, 124
Postoperative care, 133–9
  following arthroplasty, 127
  following extramedullary fixation, 84–5
  following internal fixation of intracapsular
      fracture, 56–7
  following intramedullary fixation, 107
  further fracture prevention, 138–9
Prophylaxis:
  antithrombotic, 34–5

Prophylaxis—*cont.*
  antibiotic, 35–7
Prosthesis loosening, 20, 129
Pyrexia, postoperative, 136

Reduction *see* Fracture reduction
Renal function, 22, 29, 134
Respiratory function, 29, 134–5
Reversed fracture line, 81–2
Rheumatoid arthritis, 22, 32
Richard intramedullary hip screw, 24
Richards reconstruction nail, 24
Russel-Taylor nail, 97, 102, 103

Seinsheimer classification system, 14–15
Sepsis *see* infection
Side plate:
  extramedullary fixation, 71–3
    Medoff sliding plate, 77
    short barrel plate, 75
    trochanteric stabilizing plate, 77
Silk approach, 65
Smith-Petersen approach, 114
Smith-Peterson nail, 46
Southern approach *see* Posterior approach
Static extramedullary implants, 22–3
Stracathro approach, 115
Subcapital fractures *see* Intracapsular
    fractures
Subtrochanteric fractures:
  classification of, 13–15
  extramedullary fixation, 22–4, 83–5
  intramedullary fixation, 24, 91–3
  treatment options, 23–5
  see also Extramedullary fixation
Surgical approach:
  arthroplasty, 113–16
  extramedullary fixation, 65–6
  silk approach, 65
  see also Anterolateral approach; Posterior
      approach

Thompson prosthesis, 120, 121–2
Thrombotic complications, 31, 138
  prophylaxis, 34–5
Thyroid function, 30
Timing of surgery, 33–4
  intracapsular fracture, 45–6

Total hip replacement, 112
Traction:
    preoperative, 33
Traction table *see* Fracture table
Transcervical fractures, 11
Transgluteal approach *see* Anterolateral
    approach
Treatment of extracapsular fractures, 24–5
Trochanteric fractures, 4
    classification of, 13–15
    types of, 80–82
    see also Extramedullary fixation
Trochanteric stabilizing plate, 76

Ullevaal screws, 50, 53
Undisplaced fractures:
    extracapsular, 15, 78
    intracapsular, 11
        conservative treatment, 18
        internal fixation, 18, 19

Undisplaced fractures—*cont.*
    intracapsular—*cont.*
        timing of surgery, 45
Uppsala screws, 50
Urinary tract infection, 137

Vari-Wall reconstruction nail, 24, 98, 102
Vitamin D, 2, 4, 139
von Bahr screws, 50

Warfarin, 35
Weight-bearing, 56–7, 84, 107, 126
Whittaker classification, 125
Wound closure:
    arthroplasty, 125–6
    extramedullary fixation, 73–4
    intramedullary fixation, 106
Wound infection, 136–7

Zickel classification system, 14
Zickel nail, 24, 91–2, 97

290797 W.M.D.